# THE PORTABLE BLENDER
# SMOOTHIE
## RECIPE BOOK

*Sophia Hobbs*

# CONTENTS

# CONTENTS

**Everybody loves a smoothie! Whether you drink them to hit your daily fruit and veg quota, as a pre/post gym shake, as part of a diet or just because they taste great, there are endless flavors and blends to suit your taste, lifestyle and goals.**

The technology and power of kitchen appliances have evolved to now deliver truly portable and personal blending on-the-go. Portable blenders for smoothies are powerful devices that charge via a USB cable and can be taken anywhere – office, gym, park, road-trip – the possibilities are endless. They are compact enough to fit in a bag and can be blended in any location. You can blend and drink from the same cup making these a game-changer for anyone who is busy or active and loves their smoothies whenever and wherever.

My collection of smoothies has been specially created for portable and personal blenders as opposed to larger kitchen multi-function blenders. The quantities, measurements and ingredients have all been developed to work perfectly in a smaller portable blender and for single-serving drinks. Some have as little as 3 ingredients and so can be super-simple to make. The ratio of liquids, solids and frozen ingredients will deliver a perfect smoothie every time. If you follow the ingredients, you won't overfill or block the blades and the balance of flavors is just right.

I really love simple kitchen devices which focus on one function and my recipes compliment this by being easy-to-follow and laid out in a simple, fuss-free format. All use UK measurements and ingredients easily sourced from UK supermarkets. Some foods may be easier to source in-season and you may have to search to locate some of the suggested nut-based milks, however in every case a substitute can be used.

> *It is important to note that a large proportion of my smoothies use nut milks e.g. almond milk and often nut butters so anyone who suffers from allergies or is in contact with a sufferer should carefully read the ingredients and use substitutes where appropriate.*

All the recipes in this book have been tested using a **Ninja Blast Portable Blender** and a **CobocenPortable Mini Blender**. Both these devices use a larger cup size between 570-600ml and have a maximum fill capacity for ingredients of 470ml. *My recipes are not suitable for blenders that use smaller cup sizes of between 380ml-420ml* and ingredients would therefore need to be adjusted accordingly.

While all my recipes are easy-to-follow, there are some important points you must stick to if you want to create the perfect smoothie every time:

- Read and follow the manufacturer's instructions for your blender.
- Make sure that your blender is fully charged before use. A full charge can take up to 2hrs so plan ahead.
- Familiarize yourself with the troubleshooting process for your device e.g. warning light sequence for blocked blades or charge status.
- Add the ingredients in the order listed in the recipe, always starting with liquids and ending with frozen ingredients. Note the minimum liquid level in some devices.

- Never exceed the max fill line. You can use a wooden spoon to push the ingredients down into the cup if needed.
- Don't be tempted to use more of any one ingredient in a recipe as this will make a difference to the overall capacity that your device can adequately handle both in terms of max fill and the blender's capability to crush frozen ingredients. For example, you may be tempted to include 100g of frozen fruit instead of the recommended *75g*. Your blender may struggle to blast through the additional quantity in relation to the liquid ingredients. This may cause the blending process to stop and will affect the consistency of the smoothie.
- It is perfectly acceptable to shake and tilt the blender to move stuck ingredients.
- Leafy greens can be scrunched up or chopped prior to placing in the cup so they take up less space. *For reference, a handful refers to approximately 15g.*
- Firmer vegetables like carrot and beetroot should be chopped into small pieces (*approx. 2.5cm*) to allow the blades to blend.
- Where recipes include ice cubes, the size is based on an average cube from a home-freezer ice tray. Larger varieties bought from a supermarket may struggle in a portable blender. Remember do not over-fill!

For best results follow these steps when adding ingredients
to your portable blender:

| | |
|---|---|
| → | Start with liquid ingredients |
| → | Followed by fresh fruit |
| → | Any leafy greens |
| → | Dry and sticky ingredients including protein powders and honey/maple syrup |
| → | Frozen ingredients |

Max Fill
Frozen Ingredients
Dry & Sticky Ingredients
Leafy Greens
Fresh Fruit
Liquids

Recipes are collected into the following sections:

| | |
|---|---|
| → | Everyday Classic Smoothies |
| → | Morning Smoothies – **great for a pick-up** |
| → | Protein Smoothies & Shakes – **perfect for pre & post workouts** |
| → | Lunchtime smoothies – **filling and great to get you through the day** |
| → | Green Smoothies – **healthy, nutritious & vibrant** |
| → | Vegan & Dairy Free Smoothies |
| → | Frozen Slushies – **fun and extra-cold** |
| → | Gut Health Smoothies – **probiotic goodness for your gut** |

**Perfect, portable and personal smoothies packed with flavor. I hope you enjoy making them and feel free to experiment with your own blends and inventions – the possibilities are endless.**

# CLASSIC STRAWBERRY SMOOTHIE

## Ingredients

→ **1 CUP WHOLE MILK**

→ **½ TSP VANILLA EXTRACT**

→ **1 CUP FROZEN STRAWBERRIES**

## Method

**↓ONE**
Ensure the motor base is fully charged. Install the blender cup on the base securely, then power on.

**↓TWO**
Add all the ingredients to the cup in **the order listed** (liquids followed by solids) ensuring the **max fill** line is not exceeded.

**↓THREE**
Secure the lid to the blender cup.

**↓FOUR**
Start the blending process. If necessary, repeat the blending process until completely smooth.

**↓FIVE**
Sip from the cup or pour into a glass and enjoy!

### Nutrition
CALORIES: 160
PROTEIN: 8G
TOTAL FAT: 5G
SATURATED FAT: 3G
CARBS: 22G
FIBER: 2G
SUGARS: 19G

SERVES

1

# CHEERFUL CHERRY SMOOTHIE

## Ingredients

→ **1 CUP UNSWEETENED ALMOND MILK**

→ **½ SMALL BANANA, CHOPPED**

→ **1 TBSP CHIA SEEDS**

→ **½ CUP FROZEN CHERRIES**

## Method

**↓ONE**
Ensure the motor base is fully charged. Install the blender cup on the base securely, then power on.

**↓TWO**
Add all the ingredients to the cup in **the order listed** (liquids followed by solids) ensuring the **max fill** line is not exceeded.

**↓THREE**
Secure the lid to the blender cup.

**↓FOUR**
Start the blending process. If necessary, repeat the blending process until completely smooth.

**↓FIVE**
Sip from the cup or pour into a glass and enjoy!

### Nutrition

CALORIES: 170
PROTEIN: 4G
TOTAL FAT: 4G
SATURATED FAT: 0G
CARBS: 30G
FIBER: 8G
SUGARS: 17G

SERVES

1

# KIWI COOLER SMOOTHIE

## Ingredients

→ ¾ **CUP UNSWEETENED COCONUT MILK**

→ **1 TBSP LIME JUICE**

→ **2 KIWI FRUITS, PEELED & CHOPPED**

→ **½ SMALL BANANA, CHOPPED**

→ **½ CUP FROZEN MANGO CHUNKS**

## Method

**↓ONE**
Ensure the motor base is fully charged. Install the blender cup on the base securely, then power on.

**↓TWO**
Add all the ingredients to the cup in **the order listed** (liquids followed by solids) ensuring the **max fill** line is not exceeded.

**↓THREE**
Secure the lid to the blender cup.

**↓FOUR**
Start the blending process. If necessary, repeat the blending process until completely smooth.

**↓FIVE**
Sip from the cup or pour into a glass and enjoy!

### Nutrition
CALORIES: 200
PROTEIN: 3G
TOTAL FAT: 1G
SATURATED FAT: 0G
CARBS: 47G
FIBER: 6G
SUGARS: 36G

SERVES

1

# TRIPLE BERRY BLAST

## Ingredients

→ **1 CUP UNSWEETENED OAT MILK**

→ **⅓ CUP FROZEN RASPBERRIES**

→ **⅓ CUP FROZEN BLUEBERRIES**

→ **⅓ CUP FROZEN BLACKBERRIES**

## Method

**↓ONE**
Ensure the motor base is fully charged. Install the blender cup on the base securely, then power on.

**↓TWO**
Add all the ingredients to the cup in **the order listed** (liquids followed by solids) ensuring the **max fill** line is not exceeded.

**↓THREE**
Secure the lid to the blender cup.

**↓FOUR**
Start the blending process. If necessary, repeat the blending process until completely smooth.

**↓FIVE**
Sip from the cup or pour into a glass and enjoy!

### Nutrition

CALORIES: 120
PROTEIN: 4G
TOTAL FAT: 2.5G
SATURATED FAT: 0G
CARBS: 22G
FIBER: 5G
SUGARS: 12G

SERVES

1

# RASPBERRY RIPPLE SMOOTHIE

## Ingredients

→ **1 CUP WHOLE MILK**

→ **½ CUP PLAIN GREEK YOGURT**

→ **½ CUP FROZEN RASPBERRIES**

### Nutrition

CALORIES: 250
PROTEIN: 17G
TOTAL FAT: 8G
SATURATED FAT: 5G
CARBS: 28G
FIBER: 5G
SUGARS: 24G

SERVES

## Method

**↓ONE**
Ensure the motor base is fully charged. Install the blender cup on the base securely, then power on.

**↓TWO**
Add all the ingredients to the cup in **the order listed** (liquids followed by solids) ensuring the **max fill** line is not exceeded.

**↓THREE**
Secure the lid to the blender cup.

**↓FOUR**
Start the blending process. If necessary, repeat the blending process until completely smooth.

**↓FIVE**
Sip from the cup or pour into a glass and enjoy!

# PINEAPPLE CUCUMBER REFRESHER

## Ingredients

→ **¾ CUP UNSWEETENED COCONUT MILK**

→ **1 TBSP LIME JUICE**

→ **⅓ CUCUMBER, CHOPPED**

→ **½ CUP PINEAPPLE CHUNKS**

→ **2-3 ICE CUBES**

## Method

**↓ONE**
Ensure the motor base is fully charged. Install the blender cup on the base securely, then power on.

**↓TWO**
Add all the ingredients to the cup in **the order listed** (liquids followed by solids) ensuring the **max fill** line is not exceeded.

**↓THREE**
Secure the lid to the blender cup.

**↓FOUR**
Start the blending process. If necessary, repeat the blending process until completely smooth.

**↓FIVE**
Sip from the cup or pour into a glass and enjoy!

### Nutrition

CALORIES: 80
PROTEIN: 1G
TOTAL FAT: 0G
SATURATED FAT: 0G
CARBS: 19G
FIBER: 2G
SUGARS: 15G

**SERVES**

1

# SUNSHINE SUMMER SMOOTHIE

## Ingredients

→ **1 CUP ORANGE JUICE**

→ **½ SMALL BANANA, CHOPPED**

→ **1 TBSP CHIA SEEDS**

→ **⅓ CUP FROZEN MANGO CHUNKS**

→ **¾ CUP FROZEN PEACH SLICES**

### Nutrition ~

**CALORIES: 240**
**PROTEIN: 4G**
**TOTAL FAT: 4G**
**SATURATED FAT: 0G**
**CARBS: 52G**
**FIBER: 8G**
**SUGARS: 41G**

**SERVES**

## Method

**↓ONE**
Ensure the motor base is fully charged. Install the blender cup on the base securely, then power on.

**↓TWO**
Add all the ingredients to the cup in **the order listed** (liquids followed by solids) ensuring the **max fill** line is not exceeded.

**↓THREE**
Secure the lid to the blender cup.

**↓FOUR**
Start the blending process. If necessary, repeat the blending process until completely smooth.

**↓FIVE**
Sip from the cup or pour into a glass and enjoy!

# TROPICAL PARADISE

## Ingredients

→ **¾ CUP UNSWEETENED COCONUT MILK**

→ **⅔ CUP MANGO FLESH, PITTED AND CHOPPED**

→ **¾ CUP PAPAYA FLESH, CUBED, SEEDS DISCARDED**

→ **⅓ SMALL BANANA, CHOPPED**

### Nutrition

**CALORIES: 255**
**PROTEIN: 3G**
**TOTAL FAT: 8G**
**SATURATED FAT: 7G**
**CARBS: 49G**
**FIBER: 5G**
**SUGARS: 39G**

**SERVES**

**1**

## Method

**↓ONE**
Ensure the motor base is fully charged. Install the blender cup on the base securely, then power on.

**↓TWO**
Add all the ingredients to the cup in **the order listed** (liquids followed by solids) ensuring the **max fill** line is not exceeded.

**↓THREE**
Secure the lid to the blender cup.

**↓FOUR**
Start the blending process. If necessary, repeat the blending process until completely smooth.

**↓FIVE**
Sip from the cup or pour into a glass and enjoy!

# PEACH MANGO MELODY

## Ingredients

→ **1 CUP WHOLE MILK**

→ **¾ CUP FROZEN PEACH SLICES**

→ **½ CUP FROZEN MANGO CHUNKS**

## Method

**↓ONE**
Ensure the motor base is fully charged. Install the blender cup on the base securely, then power on.

**↓TWO**
Add all the ingredients to the cup in **the order listed** (liquids followed by solids) ensuring the **max fill** line is not exceeded.

**↓THREE**
Secure the lid to the blender cup.

**↓FOUR**
Start the blending process. If necessary, repeat the blending process until completely smooth.

**↓FIVE**
Sip from the cup or pour into a glass and enjoy!

### Nutrition
CALORIES: 220
PROTEIN: 8G
TOTAL FAT: 5G
SATURATED FAT: 3G
CARBS: 39G
FIBER: 4G
SUGARS: 34G

**SERVES**

1

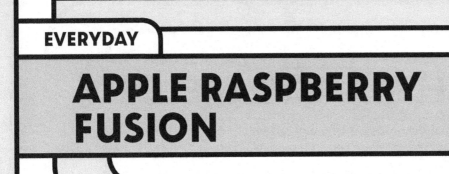

# APPLE RASPBERRY FUSION

## Ingredients

→ **1 CUP UNSWEETENED APPLE JUICE**

→ **1 RED APPLE, CORED & CHOPPED**

→ **1 TBSP GROUND FLAXSEED**

→ **½ CUP FROZEN RASPBERRIES**

## Method

**↓ONE**
Ensure the motor base is fully charged. Install the blender cup on the base securely, then power on.

**↓TWO**
Add all the ingredients to the cup in **the order listed** (liquids followed by solids) ensuring the **max fill** line is not exceeded.

**↓THREE**
Secure the lid to the blender cup.

**↓FOUR**
Start the blending process. If necessary, repeat the blending process until completely smooth.

**↓FIVE**
Sip from the cup or pour into a glass and enjoy!

### Nutrition ~

CALORIES: 210
PROTEIN: 3G
TOTAL FAT: 3G
SATURATED FAT: 0G
CARBS: 46G
FIBER: 9G
SUGARS: 33G

**SERVES**

1

# MORNING MOCHA KICK

## Ingredients

→ **1 CUP UNSWEETENED ALMOND MILK**

→ **½ CUP COLD BREW COFFEE**

→ **1 TBSP COCOA POWDER**

→ **2 TBSP ALMOND BUTTER**

→ **½ TSP VANILLA EXTRACT**

→ **½ SMALL FROZEN BANANA, CHOPPED**

### Nutrition

**CALORIES:** 280
**PROTEIN:** 7G
**TOTAL FAT:** 20G
**SATURATED FAT:** 1.5G
**CARBS:** 22G
**FIBER:** 6G
**SUGARS:** 10G

SERVES

## Method

**↓ONE**
Ensure the motor base is fully charged. Install the blender cup on the base securely, then power on.

**↓TWO**
Add all the ingredients to the cup in **the order listed** (liquids followed by solids) ensuring the **max fill** line is not exceeded.

**↓THREE**
Secure the lid to the blender cup.

**↓FOUR**
Start the blending process. If necessary, repeat the blending process until completely smooth.

**↓FIVE**
Sip from the cup or pour into a glass and enjoy!

# TROPICAL WAKE-UP CALL

## Ingredients

→ **1 CUP UNSWEETENED COCONUT MILK**

→ **1 TBSP SHREDDED COCONUT**

→ **1 TBSP FRESHLY GRATED GINGER**

→ **⅓ CUP PINEAPPLE CHUNKS**

→ **⅔ CUP FROZEN MANGO CHUNKS**

## Method

**↓ONE**
Ensure the motor base is fully charged. Install the blender cup on the base securely, then power on.

**↓TWO**
Add all the ingredients to the cup in **the order listed** (liquids followed by solids) ensuring the **max fill** line is not exceeded.

**↓THREE**
Secure the lid to the blender cup.

**↓FOUR**
Start the blending process. If necessary, repeat the blending process until completely smooth.

**↓FIVE**
Sip from the cup or pour into a glass and enjoy!

### Nutrition

CALORIES: 160
PROTEIN: 2G
TOTAL FAT: 5G
SATURATED FAT: 3.5G
CARBS: 28G
FIBER: 4G
SUGARS: 20G

SERVES

1

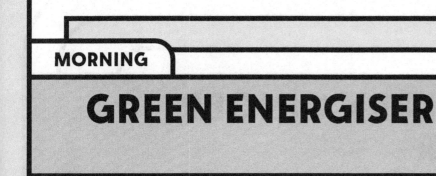

# GREEN ENERGISER

## Ingredients

→ **1 CUP UNSWEETENED COCONUT MILK**

→ **½ GREEN APPLE, CORED & CHOPPED**

→ **1 TBSP LEMON JUICE**

→ **½ TSP MATCHA POWDER**

→ **HANDFUL BABY SPINACH LEAVES**

→ **½ SMALL FROZEN BANANA, CHOPPED**

## Method

**↓ONE**
Ensure the motor base is fully charged. Install the blender cup on the base securely, then power on.

**↓TWO**
Add all the ingredients to the cup in **the order listed** (liquids followed by solids) ensuring the **max fill** line is not exceeded.

**↓THREE**
Secure the lid to the blender cup.

**↓FOUR**
Start the blending process. If necessary, repeat the blending process until completely smooth.

**↓FIVE**
Sip from the cup or pour into a glass and enjoy!

### Nutrition
**CALORIES:** 175
**PROTEIN:** 3G
**TOTAL FAT:** 5G
**SATURATED FAT:** 4.5G
**CARBS:** 33G
**FIBER:** 5G
**SUGARS:** 21G

**SERVES**

1

19

# BLUEBERRY GINGER ZINGER

## Ingredients

→ **1 CUP UNSWEETENED OAT MILK**

→ **1 TBSP FRESH GINGER, GRATED**

→ **1 TBSP LEMON JUICE**

→ **1 TSP HONEY**

→ **1 CUP FROZEN BLUEBERRIES**

## Method

**↓ONE**
Ensure the motor base is fully charged. Install the blender cup on the base securely, then power on.

**↓TWO**
Add all the ingredients to the cup in **the order listed** (liquids followed by solids) ensuring the **max fill** line is not exceeded.

**↓THREE**
Secure the lid to the blender cup.

**↓FOUR**
Start the blending process. If necessary, repeat the blending process until completely smooth.

**↓FIVE**
Sip from the cup or pour into a glass and enjoy!

### Nutrition ~

CALORIES: 165
PROTEIN: 3G
TOTAL FAT: 4G
SATURATED FAT: 0.1G
CARBS: 33G
FIBER: 5G
SUGARS: 17G

SERVES

1

20

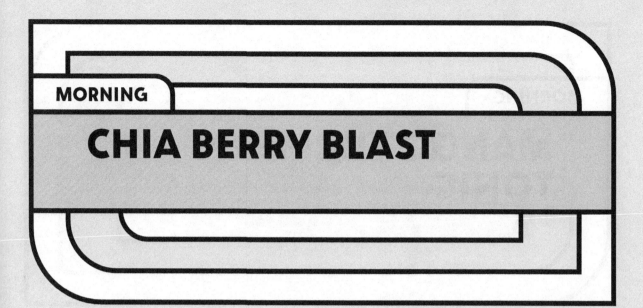

# CHIA BERRY BLAST

## Ingredients

→ **1 CUP UNSWEETENED SOYA MILK**

→ **2 TBSP CHIA SEEDS**

→ **1 CUP FROZEN MIXED BERRIES**

## Method

**↓ONE**
Ensure the motor base is fully charged. Install the blender cup on the base securely, then power on.

**↓TWO**
Add all the ingredients to the cup in **the order listed** (liquids followed by solids) ensuring the **max fill** line is not exceeded.

**↓THREE**
Secure the lid to the blender cup.

**↓FOUR**
Start the blending process. If necessary, repeat the blending process until completely smooth.

**↓FIVE**
Sip from the cup or pour into a glass and enjoy!

### Nutrition
CALORIES: 220
PROTEIN: 10G
TOTAL FAT: 9G
SATURATED FAT: 1G
CARBS: 26G
FIBER: 14G
SUGARS: 11G

**SERVES**

1

# MANGO TURMERIC TONIC

## Ingredients

→ **1 CUP UNSWEETENED ALMOND MILK**

→ **½ TSP GROUND TURMERIC**

→ **1 CUP FROZEN MANGO CHUNKS**

## Method

**↓ONE**
Ensure the motor base is fully charged. Install the blender cup on the base securely, then power on.

**↓TWO**
Add all the ingredients to the cup in **the order listed** (liquids followed by solids) ensuring the **max fill** line is not exceeded.

**↓THREE**
Secure the lid to the blender cup.

**↓FOUR**
Start the blending process. If necessary, repeat the blending process until completely smooth.

**↓FIVE**
Sip from the cup or pour into a glass and enjoy!

### Nutrition ~

CALORIES: 130
PROTEIN: 2G
TOTAL FAT: 4G
SATURATED FAT: 0G
CARBS: 22G
FIBER: 3G
SUGARS: 16G

SERVES

1

# MATCHA MINT COOLER

## Ingredients

→ **1 CUP UNSWEETENED COCONUT MILK**

→ **1 TBSP LEMON JUICE**

→ **1 TSP MATCHA POWDER**

→ **10 FRESH MINT LEAVES**

→ **⅔ CUP FROZEN PINEAPPLE CHUNKS**

## Method

**↓ONE**
Ensure the motor base is fully charged. Install the blender cup on the base securely, then power on.

**↓TWO**
Add all the ingredients to the cup in **the order listed** (liquids followed by solids) ensuring the **max fill** line is not exceeded.

**↓THREE**
Secure the lid to the blender cup.

**↓FOUR**
Start the blending process. If necessary, repeat the blending process until completely smooth.

**↓FIVE**
Sip from the cup or pour into a glass and enjoy!

### Nutrition

**CALORIES:** 220
**PROTEIN:** 4G
**TOTAL FAT:** 14G
**SATURATED FAT:** 12G
**CARBS:** 28G
**FIBER:** 3G
**SUGARS:** 20G

**SERVES**

**1**

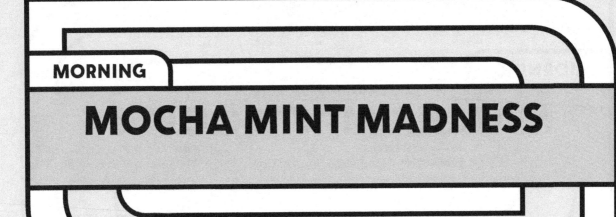

# MOCHA MINT MADNESS

## Ingredients

→ **1 CUP UNSWEETENED OAT MILK**

→ **½ CUP CHILLED COFFEE**

→ **2 TSP COCOA POWDER**

→ **10 FRESH MINT LEAVES**

→ **1 SMALL FROZEN BANANA, CHOPPED**

## Method

**↓ONE**
Ensure the motor base is fully charged. Install the blender cup on the base securely, then power on.

**↓TWO**
Add all the ingredients to the cup in **the order listed** (liquids followed by solids) ensuring the **max fill** line is not exceeded.

**↓THREE**
Secure the lid to the blender cup.

**↓FOUR**
Start the blending process. If necessary, repeat the blending process until completely smooth.

**↓FIVE**
Sip from the cup or pour into a glass and enjoy!

### Nutrition

CALORIES: 186
PROTEIN: 5G
TOTAL FAT: 4G
SATURATED FAT: 0.7G
CARBS: 35G
FIBER: 6G
SUGARS: 16G

SERVES

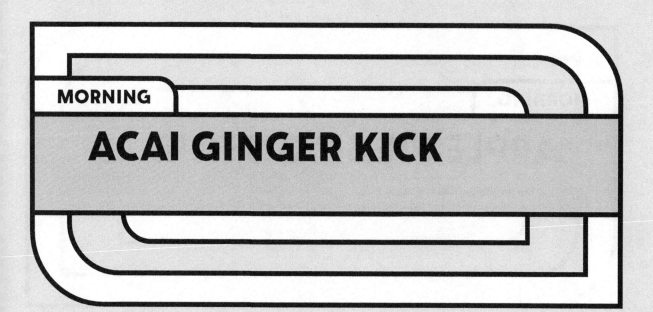

# ACAI GINGER KICK

## Ingredients

→ **1 CUP UNSWEETENED SOY MILK**

→ **1 TBSP LIME JUICE**

→ **1 TBSP ACAI POWDER**

→ **1 TBSP FRESHLY GRATED GINGER**

→ **½ CUP FROZEN MIXED BERRIES**

## Method

**↓ONE**
Ensure the motor base is fully charged. Install the blender cup on the base securely, then power on.

**↓TWO**
Add all the ingredients to the cup in **the order listed** (liquids followed by solids) ensuring the **max fill** line is not exceeded.

**↓THREE**
Secure the lid to the blender cup.

**↓FOUR**
Start the blending process. If necessary, repeat the blending process until completely smooth.

**↓FIVE**
Sip from the cup or pour into a glass and enjoy!

### Nutrition
CALORIES: 170
PROTEIN: 7G
TOTAL FAT: 4G
SATURATED FAT: 0.5G
CARBS: 26G
FIBER: 8G
SUGARS: 14G

**SERVES**

1

# APPLE PIE SMOOTHIE

## Ingredients

→ **1 CUP UNSWEETENED ALMOND MILK**

→ **½ TSP GROUND NUTMEG**

→ **1 TSP GROUND CINNAMON**

→ **1 GREEN APPLE, CORED & CHOPPED**

→ **½ SMALL FROZEN BANANA, CHOPPED**

### Nutrition
CALORIES: 180
PROTEIN: 3G
TOTAL FAT: 4G
SATURATED FAT: 0G
CARBS: 35G
FIBER: 7G
SUGARS: 20G

**SERVES**

**1**

## Method

**↓ONE**
Ensure the motor base is fully charged. Install the blender cup on the base securely, then power on.

**↓TWO**
Add all the ingredients to the cup in **the order listed** (liquids followed by solids) ensuring the **max fill** line is not exceeded.

**↓THREE**
Secure the lid to the blender cup.

**↓FOUR**
Start the blending process. If necessary, repeat the blending process until completely smooth.

**↓FIVE**
Sip from the cup or pour into a glass and enjoy!

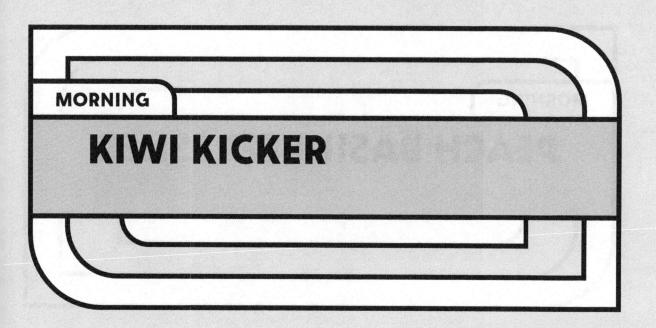

# KIWI KICKER

## Ingredients

→ **¾ CUP COCONUT WATER**

→ **1 TBSP LIME JUICE**

→ **1 TSP FRESHLY GRATED GINGER**

→ **2 KIWI FRUITS, PEELED & CHOPPED**

→ **⅓ CUP FROZEN MANGO CHUNKS**

## Method

**↓ONE**
Ensure the motor base is fully charged. Install the blender cup on the base securely, then power on.

**↓TWO**
Add all the ingredients to the cup in **the order listed** (liquids followed by solids) ensuring the **max fill** line is not exceeded.

**↓THREE**
Secure the lid to the blender cup.

**↓FOUR**
Start the blending process. If necessary, repeat the blending process until completely smooth.

**↓FIVE**
Sip from the cup or pour into a glass and enjoy!

### Nutrition
CALORIES: 140
PROTEIN: 2G
TOTAL FAT: 1G
SATURATED FAT: 0G
CARBS: 33G
FIBER: 5G
SUGARS: 20G

**SERVES**

1

# PEACH BASIL REFRESHER

## Ingredients

→ **1 CUP UNSWEETENED COCONUT WATER**

→ **5-6 FRESH BASIL LEAVES**

→ **1 TBSP LIME JUICE**

→ **1 TSP HONEY**

→ **½ CUP FROZEN PEACH SLICES**

## Method

**↓ONE**
Ensure the motor base is fully charged. Install the blender cup on the base securely, then power on.

**↓TWO**
Add all the ingredients to the cup in **the order listed** (liquids followed by solids) ensuring the **max fill** line is not exceeded.

**↓THREE**
Secure the lid to the blender cup.

**↓FOUR**
Start the blending process. If necessary, repeat the blending process until completely smooth.

**↓FIVE**
Sip from the cup or pour into a glass and enjoy!

### Nutrition ~

**CALORIES:** 70
**PROTEIN:** 1G
**TOTAL FAT:** 0G
**SATURATED FAT:** 0G
**CARBS:** 17G
**FIBER:** 2G
**SUGARS:** 15G

**SERVES**

1

# GUARANA GRAPE KICK

## Ingredients

→ **1 CUP UNSWEETENED OAT MILK**

→ **⅓ CUP ROLLED OATS**

→ **1 TSP GUARANA POWDER**

→ **⅔ CUP FROZEN RED GRAPES**

### Nutrition
CALORIES: 290
PROTEIN: 10G
TOTAL FAT: 6G
SATURATED FAT: 1G
CARBS: 53G
FIBER: 7G
SUGARS: 20G

**SERVES**

**1**

## Method

**↓ONE**
Ensure the motor base is fully charged. Install the blender cup on the base securely, then power on.

**↓TWO**
Add all the ingredients to the cup in **the order listed** (liquids followed by solids) ensuring the **max fill** line is not exceeded.

**↓THREE**
Secure the lid to the blender cup.

**↓FOUR**
Start the blending process. If necessary, repeat the blending process until completely smooth.

**↓FIVE**
Sip from the cup or pour into a glass and enjoy!

# CHOCOLATE CHERRY BOMB

## Ingredients

→ **1 CUP UNSWEETENED SOY MILK**

→ **2 TSP COCOA POWDER**

→ **⅔ CUP FROZEN PITTED CHERRIES**

→ **2-3 ICE CUBES**

## Method

**↓ONE**
Ensure the motor base is fully charged. Install the blender cup on the base securely, then power on.

**↓TWO**
Add all the ingredients to the cup in **the order listed** (liquids followed by solids) ensuring the **max fill** line is not exceeded.

**↓THREE**
Secure the lid to the blender cup.

**↓FOUR**
Start the blending process. If necessary, repeat the blending process until completely smooth.

**↓FIVE**
Sip from the cup or pour into a glass and enjoy!

### Nutrition
CALORIES: 150
PROTEIN: 8G
TOTAL FAT: 4G
SATURATED FAT: 0.5G
CARBS: 22G
FIBER: 5G
SUGARS: 16G

SERVES

1

# PINA COLADA SMOOTHIE

## Ingredients

→ **½ CUP UNSWEETENED COCONUT MILK**

→ **1 TBSP LIME JUICE**

→ **2 TBSP SHREDDED COCONUT**

→ **⅔ CUP FROZEN PINEAPPLE CHUNKS**

### Nutrition

CALORIES: 205
PROTEIN: 2G
TOTAL FAT: 12G
SATURATED FAT: 11G
CARBS: 25G
FIBER: 4G
SUGARS: 17G

SERVES

## Method

**↓ONE**
Ensure the motor base is fully charged. Install the blender cup on the base securely, then power on.

**↓TWO**
Add all the ingredients to the cup in **the order listed** (liquids followed by solids) ensuring the **max fill** line is not exceeded.

**↓THREE**
Secure the lid to the blender cup.

**↓FOUR**
Start the blending process. If necessary, repeat the blending process until completely smooth.

**↓FIVE**
Sip from the cup or pour into a glass and enjoy!

# STRAWBERRY LEMON SLAM

## Ingredients

→ **1 CUP UNSWEETENED ALMOND MILK**

→ **1 TBSP LEMON JUICE**

→ **⅔ CUP FROZEN STRAWBERRIES**

→ **⅔ ICE CUBES**

## Method

**↓ONE**
Ensure the motor base is fully charged. Install the blender cup on the base securely, then power on.

**↓TWO**
Add all the ingredients to the cup in **the order listed** (liquids followed by solids) ensuring the **max fill** line is not exceeded.

**↓THREE**
Secure the lid to the blender cup.

**↓FOUR**
Start the blending process. If necessary, repeat the blending process until completely smooth.

**↓FIVE**
Sip from the cup or pour into a glass and enjoy!

### Nutrition
CALORIES: 90
PROTEIN: 2G
TOTAL FAT: 3G
SATURATED FAT: 0G
CARBS: 15G
FIBER: 4G
SUGARS: 10G

SERVES

**1**

## MORNING

# CACAO AVOCADO POWER

## Ingredients

→ **1 CUP UNSWEETENED COCONUT MILK**

→ **½ RIPE AVOCADO, PITTED**

→ **½ TSP VANILLA EXTRACT**

→ **1 TBSP CACAO POWDER**

## Method

**↓ONE**
Ensure the motor base is fully charged. Install the blender cup on the base securely, then power on.

**↓TWO**
Add all the ingredients to the cup in **the order listed** (liquids followed by solids) ensuring the **max fill** line is not exceeded.

**↓THREE**
Secure the lid to the blender cup.

**↓FOUR**
Start the blending process. If necessary, repeat the blending process until completely smooth.

**↓FIVE**
Sip from the cup or pour into a glass and enjoy!

### Nutrition

CALORIES: 225
PROTEIN: 4G
TOTAL FAT: 18G
SATURATED FAT: 3G
CARBS: 17G
FIBER: 11G
SUGARS: 4G

SERVES

1

# BEET BERRY ENERGISER

## Ingredients

→ **1 CUP UNSWEETENED OAT MILK**

→ **1 TBSP GROUND FLAXSEED**

→ **1 SMALL BEET, PEELED AND CHOPPED**

→ **½ CUP FROZEN MIXED BERRIES**

## Method

**↓ONE**
Ensure the motor base is fully charged. Install the blender cup on the base securely, then power on.

**↓TWO**
Add all the ingredients to the cup in **the order listed** (liquids followed by solids) ensuring the **max fill** line is not exceeded.

**↓THREE**
Secure the lid to the blender cup.

**↓FOUR**
Start the blending process. If necessary, repeat the blending process until completely smooth.

**↓FIVE**
Sip from the cup or pour into a glass and enjoy!

### Nutrition
CALORIES: 240
PROTEIN: 7G
TOTAL FAT: 7G
SATURATED FAT: 1G
CARBS: 37G
FIBER: 10G
SUGARS: 15G

SERVES

1

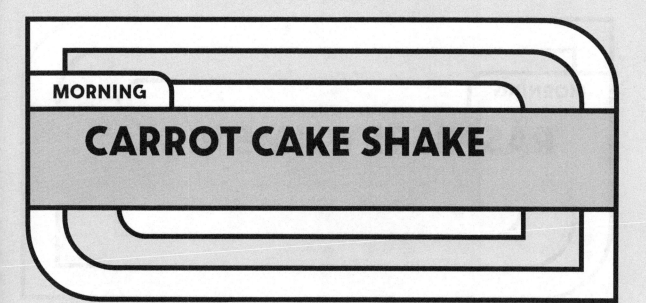

# CARROT CAKE SHAKE

## Ingredients

→ **1 CUP UNSWEETENED SOY MILK**

→ **½ TSP GROUND CINNAMON**

→ **2 TBSP ROLLED OATS**

→ **1 MEDIUM CARROT, PEELED AND CHOPPED**

→ **½ SMALL FROZEN BANANA, CHOPPED**

## Method

### ↓ONE
Ensure the motor base is fully charged. Install the blender cup on the base securely, then power on.

### ↓TWO
Add all the ingredients to the cup in **the order listed** (liquids followed by solids) ensuring the **max fill** line is not exceeded.

### ↓THREE
Secure the lid to the blender cup.

### ↓FOUR
Start the blending process. If necessary, repeat the blending process until completely smooth.

### ↓FIVE
Sip from the cup or pour into a glass and enjoy!

### Nutrition

CALORIES: 230
PROTEIN: 9G
TOTAL FAT: 6G
SATURATED FAT: 1G
CARBS: 35G
FIBER: 7G
SUGARS: 16G

SERVES

1

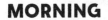

# RASPBERRY LIME RICKEY

## Ingredients

→ **1 CUP SPARKLING WATER**

→ **1 TBSP LIME JUICE**

→ **1 TBSP HONEY**

→ **⅔ CUP FROZEN RASPBERRIES**

→ **2-3 ICE CUBES**

### Nutrition

CALORIES: 80
PROTEIN: 1G
TOTAL FAT: 0G
SATURATED FAT: 0G
CARBS: 20G
FIBER: 5G
SUGARS: 15G

**SERVES**

## Method

**↓ONE**
Ensure the motor base is fully charged. Install the blender cup on the base securely, then power on.

**↓TWO**
Add all the ingredients to the cup in **the order listed** (liquids followed by solids) ensuring the **max fill** line is not exceeded.

**↓THREE**
Secure the lid to the blender cup.

**↓FOUR**
Start the blending process. If necessary, repeat the blending process until completely smooth.

**↓FIVE**
Sip from the cup or pour into a glass and enjoy!

# PEANUT BUTTER BANANA OAT SMOOTHIE

## Ingredients

→ **1 CUP UNSWEETENED SOY MILK**

→ **½ SMALL BANANA, CHOPPED**

→ **2 TBSP PEANUT BUTTER**

→ **1 TSP HONEY**

→ **⅓ CUP ROLLED OATS**

→ **1 TBSP CHIA SEEDS**

→ **2-3 ICE CUBES**

### Nutrition
**CALORIES:** 530
**PROTEIN:** 25G
**TOTAL FAT:** 25G
**SATURATED FAT:** 2.5G
**CARBS:** 59G
**FIBER:** 10G
**SUGARS:** 24G

**SERVES**

1

## Method

**↓ONE**
Ensure the motor base is fully charged. Install the blender cup on the base securely, then power on.

**↓TWO**
Add all the ingredients to the cup in **the order listed** (liquids followed by solids) ensuring the **max fill** line is not exceeded.

**↓THREE**
Secure the lid to the blender cup.

**↓FOUR**
Start the blending process. If necessary, repeat the blending process until completely smooth.

**↓FIVE**
Sip from the cup or pour into a glass and enjoy!

# AVOCADO SPINACH GREEK YOGHURT SMOOTHIE

## Ingredients

→ **1 CUP UNSWEETENED COCONUT MILK**

→ **⅓ CUP GREEK YOGURT**

→ **½ AVOCADO, PITTED**

→ **HANDFUL SPINACH**

→ **1 TBSP GROUND FLAXSEED**

→ **2-3 ICE CUBES**

### Nutrition

CALORIES: 395
PROTEIN: 14G
TOTAL FAT: 27G
SATURATED FAT: 11G
CARBS: 28G
FIBER: 10G
SUGARS: 11G

SERVES

## Method

**↓ONE**
Ensure the motor base is fully charged. Install the blender cup on the base securely, then power on.

**↓TWO**
Add all the ingredients to the cup in **the order listed** (liquids followed by solids) ensuring the **max fill** line is not exceeded.

**↓THREE**
Secure the lid to the blender cup.

**↓FOUR**
Start the blending process. If necessary, repeat the blending process until completely smooth.

**↓FIVE**
Sip from the cup or pour into a glass and enjoy!

# ALMOND BUTTER BERRY SMOOTHIE

## Ingredients

→ **1 CUP UNSWEETENED ALMOND MILK**

→ **2 TBSP ALMOND BUTTER**

→ **⅓ CUP ROLLED OATS**

→ **1 TBSP CHIA SEEDS**

→ **½ CUP FROZEN RASPBERRIES**

→ **½ CUP FROZEN BLUEBERRIES**

## Method

**↓ONE**
Ensure the motor base is fully charged. Install the blender cup on the base securely, then power on.

**↓TWO**
Add all the ingredients to the cup in **the order listed** (liquids followed by solids) ensuring the **max fill** line is not exceeded.

**↓THREE**
Secure the lid to the blender cup.

**↓FOUR**
Start the blending process. If necessary, repeat the blending process until completely smooth.

**↓FIVE**
Sip from the cup or pour into a glass and enjoy!

### Nutrition
CALORIES: 440
PROTEIN: 14G
TOTAL FAT: 29G
SATURATED FAT: 2G
CARBS: 38G
FIBER: 13G
SUGARS: 13G

SERVES

1

# COCONUT MANGO CHIA SMOOTHIE

## Ingredients

→ **1 CUP UNSWEETENED COCONUT MILK**

→ **½ MANGO FLESH, PITTED & CHOPPED**

→ **1 TBSP CHIA SEEDS**

→ **1 TBSP SHREDDED COCONUT**

→ **4-5 ICE CUBES**

### Nutrition ~
**CALORIES: 335**
**PROTEIN: 4G**
**TOTAL FAT: 22G**
**SATURATED FAT: 19G**
**CARBS: 38G**
**FIBER: 9G**
**SUGARS: 33G**

SERVES

**1**

## Method

**↓ONE**
Ensure the motor base is fully charged. Install the blender cup on the base securely, then power on.

**↓TWO**
Add all the ingredients to the cup in **the order listed** (liquids followed by solids) ensuring the **max fill** line is not exceeded.

**↓THREE**
Secure the lid to the blender cup.

**↓FOUR**
Start the blending process. If necessary, repeat the blending process until completely smooth.

**↓FIVE**
Sip from the cup or pour into a glass and enjoy!

# PEACH COTTAGE CHEESE SMOOTHIE

## Ingredients

→ **1 CUP UNSWEETENED OAT MILK**

→ **½ TSP VANILLA EXTRACT**

→ **½ CUP COTTAGE CHEESE**

→ **1 TBSP GROUND FLAXSEED**

→ **½ CUP FROZEN PEACH SLICES**

## Method

**↓ONE**
Ensure the motor base is fully charged. Install the blender cup on the base securely, then power on.

**↓TWO**
Add all the ingredients to the cup in **the order listed** (liquids followed by solids) ensuring the **max fill** line is not exceeded.

**↓THREE**
Secure the lid to the blender cup.

**↓FOUR**
Start the blending process. If necessary, repeat the blending process until completely smooth.

**↓FIVE**
Sip from the cup or pour into a glass and enjoy!

### Nutrition

CALORIES: 340
PROTEIN: 28G
TOTAL FAT: 12G
SATURATED FAT: 2G
CARBS: 34G
FIBER: 4G
SUGARS: 27G

SERVES

1

# BANANA NUT BUTTER SMOOTHIE

## Ingredients

→ **1 CUP UNSWEETENED ALMOND MILK**

→ **½ SMALL BANANA, CHOPPED**

→ **2 TBSP ALMOND BUTTER**

→ **¼ CUP CASHEW NUTS**

→ **1 TBSP HEMP SEEDS**

→ **1 TSP HONEY**

→ **4-5 ICE CUBES**

### Nutrition

CALORIES: 440
PROTEIN: 14G
TOTAL FAT: 35G
SATURATED FAT: 3G
CARBS: 25G
FIBER: 7G
SUGARS: 15G

SERVES

1

## Method

**↓ONE**
Ensure the motor base is fully charged. Install the blender cup on the base securely, then power on.

**↓TWO**
Add all the ingredients to the cup in **the order listed** (liquids followed by solids) ensuring the **max fill** line is not exceeded.

**↓THREE**
Secure the lid to the blender cup.

**↓FOUR**
Start the blending process. If necessary, repeat the blending process until completely smooth.

**↓FIVE**
Sip from the cup or pour into a glass and enjoy!

# PINEAPPLE SPINACH SMOOTHIE

## Ingredients

→ **1 CUP UNSWEETENED COCONUT MILK**

→ **1 TBSP LIME JUICE**

→ **HANDFUL SPINACH**

→ **1 TBSP CHIA SEEDS**

→ **1 SCOOP (30G) VANILLA PROTEIN POWDER**

→ **½ CUP FROZEN PINEAPPLE CHUNKS**

### Nutrition

CALORIES: 330
PROTEIN: 25G
TOTAL FAT: 6G
SATURATED FAT: 4G
CARBS: 42G
FIBER: 7G
SUGARS: 30G

SERVES

## Method

**↓ONE**
Ensure the motor base is fully charged. Install the blender cup on the base securely, then power on.

**↓TWO**
Add all the ingredients to the cup in **the order listed** (liquids followed by solids) ensuring the **max fill** line is not exceeded.

**↓THREE**
Secure the lid to the blender cup.

**↓FOUR**
Start the blending process. If necessary, repeat the blending process until completely smooth.

**↓FIVE**
Sip from the cup or pour into a glass and enjoy!

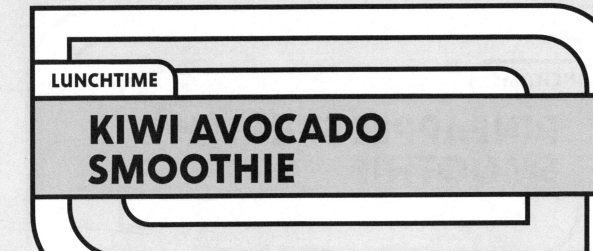

# KIWI AVOCADO SMOOTHIE

## Ingredients

→ **1 CUP UNSWEETENED SOY MILK**

→ **1 TBSP LIME JUICE**

→ **½ AVOCADO, PITTED**

→ **2 KIWIS, PEELED & CHOPPED**

→ **1 TBSP GROUND FLAXSEED**

→ **2-3 ICE CUBES**

## Method

**↓ONE**
Ensure the motor base is fully charged. Install the blender cup on the base securely, then power on.

**↓TWO**
Add all the ingredients to the cup in **the order listed** (liquids followed by solids) ensuring the **max fill** line is not exceeded.

**↓THREE**
Secure the lid to the blender cup.

**↓FOUR**
Start the blending process. If necessary, repeat the blending process until completely smooth.

**↓FIVE**
Sip from the cup or pour into a glass and enjoy!

### Nutrition

CALORIES: 390
PROTEIN: 16G
TOTAL FAT: 24G
SATURATED FAT: 2G
CARBS: 31G
FIBER: 12G
SUGARS: 20G

**SERVES**

1

# FIG ALMOND SMOOTHIE

## Ingredients

→ **1 CUP UNSWEETENED ALMOND MILK**

→ **3 DRIED FIGS, SOAKED & CHOPPED**

→ **2 TBSP ALMOND BUTTER**

→ **1 TBSP CHIA SEEDS**

→ **½ TSP GROUND CINNAMON**

→ **1 SCOOP (30G) VANILLA PROTEIN POWDER**

→ **2-3 ICE CUBES**

### Nutrition ～
**CALORIES: 570**
**PROTEIN: 28G**
**TOTAL FAT: 30G**
**SATURATED FAT: 2G**
**CARBS: 49G**
**FIBER: 14G**
**SUGARS: 29G**

**SERVES**

**1**

## Method

**↓ONE**
Ensure the motor base is fully charged. Install the blender cup on the base securely, then power on.

**↓TWO**
Add all the ingredients to the cup in **the order listed** (liquids followed by solids) ensuring the **max fill** line is not exceeded.

**↓THREE**
Secure the lid to the blender cup.

**↓FOUR**
Start the blending process. If necessary, repeat the blending process until completely smooth.

**↓FIVE**
Sip from the cup or pour into a glass and enjoy!

# PUMPKIN SEED & APPLE SMOOTHIE

## Ingredients

→ **1 CUP UNSWEETENED OAT MILK**

→ **1 GREEN APPLE, CORED & CHOPPED**

→ **2 TBSP PUMPKIN SEEDS**

→ **1 TBSP ALMOND BUTTER**

→ **½ TSP GROUND CINNAMON**

→ **½ TSP GROUND GINGER**

→ **1 TSP HONEY**

→ **½ SMALL FROZEN BANANA, CHOPPED**

### Nutrition

CALORIES: 320
PROTEIN: 8G
TOTAL FAT: 16G
SATURATED FAT: 2G
CARBS: 41G
FIBER: 8G
SUGARS: 23G

**SERVES**

1

## Method

**↓ONE**
Ensure the motor base is fully charged. Install the blender cup on the base securely, then power on.

**↓TWO**
Add all the ingredients to the cup in **the order listed** (liquids followed by solids) ensuring the **max fill** line is not exceeded.

**↓THREE**
Secure the lid to the blender cup.

**↓FOUR**
Start the blending process. If necessary, repeat the blending process until completely smooth.

**↓FIVE**
Sip from the cup or pour into a glass and enjoy!

# BANANA PEANUT SPINACH PROTEIN SMOOTHIE

## Ingredients

→ **1 CUP UNSWEETENED COCONUT MILK**

→ **½ SMALL BANANA, CHOPPED**

→ **HANDFUL SPINACH**

→ **1 TBSP PEANUT BUTTER**

→ **1 TSP CHIA SEEDS**

→ **1 TSP HONEY**

→ **1 TBSP GROUND FLAXSEED**

→ **1 SCOOP (30G) VANILLA PROTEIN POWDER**

### Nutrition

CALORIES: 470
PROTEIN: 38G
TOTAL FAT: 20G
SATURATED FAT: 5G
CARBS: 42G
FIBER: 9G
SUGARS: 23G

SERVES

## Method

**↓ONE**
Ensure the motor base is fully charged. Install the blender cup on the base securely, then power on.

**↓TWO**
Add all the ingredients to the cup in **the order listed** (liquids followed by solids) ensuring the **max fill** line is not exceeded.

**↓THREE**
Secure the lid to the blender cup.

**↓FOUR**
Start the blending process. If necessary, repeat the blending process until completely smooth.

**↓FIVE**
Sip from the cup or pour into a glass and enjoy!

# PISTACHIO DATE SMOOTHIE

## Ingredients

→ **1 CUP UNSWEETENED ALMOND MILK**

→ **3 DATES, PITTED & CHOPPED**

→ **1 TBSP ALMOND BUTTER**

→ **1 TBSP ROASTED PISTACHIOS, UNSALTED**

→ **1 TBSP CHIA SEEDS**

→ **¼ TSP GROUND CARDAMOM**

→ **4-5 ICE CUBES**

### Nutrition

CALORIES: 420
PROTEIN: 11G
TOTAL FAT: 27G
SATURATED FAT: 2G
CARBS: 41G
FIBER: 11G
SUGARS: 26G

**SERVES**

## Method

**↓ONE**
Ensure the motor base is fully charged. Install the blender cup on the base securely, then power on.

**↓TWO**
Add all the ingredients to the cup in **the order listed** (liquids followed by solids) ensuring the **max fill** line is not exceeded.

**↓THREE**
Secure the lid to the blender cup.

**↓FOUR**
Start the blending process. If necessary, repeat the blending process until completely smooth.

**↓FIVE**
Sip from the cup or pour into a glass and enjoy!

# BLUEBERRY QUINOA SMOOTHIE

## Ingredients

→ **1 CUP UNSWEETENED SOY MILK**

→ **½ SMALL BANANA, CHOPPED**

→ **2 TBSP ALMOND BUTTER**

→ **½ CUP QUINOA, COOKED**

→ **1 TBSP GROUND FLAXSEED**

→ **½ CUP FROZEN BLUEBERRIES**

### Nutrition

CALORIES: 438
PROTEIN: 19.2G
TOTAL FAT: 26.2G
SATURATED FAT: 2.3G
CARBS: 41G
FIBER: 10.2G
SUGARS: 17.1G

**SERVES**

## Method

**↓ONE**
Ensure the motor base is fully charged. Install the blender cup on the base securely, then power on.

**↓TWO**
Add all the ingredients to the cup in **the order listed** (liquids followed by solids) ensuring the **max fill** line is not exceeded.

**↓THREE**
Secure the lid to the blender cup.

**↓FOUR**
Start the blending process. If necessary, repeat the blending process until completely smooth.

**↓FIVE**
Sip from the cup or pour into a glass and enjoy!

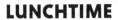

# APRICOT CASHEW SMOOTHIE

## Ingredients

→ **1 CUP UNSWEETENED OAT MILK**

→ **3 DRIED APRICOTS, SOAKED AND CHOPPED**

→ **2 TBSP CASHEW BUTTER**

→ **1 TBSP HEMP SEEDS**

→ **½ TSP GROUND GINGER**

→ **1 SCOOP (30G) VANILLA PROTEIN POWDER**

→ **4-5 ICE CUBES**

### Nutrition ~

CALORIES: 570
PROTEIN: 31G
TOTAL FAT: 29G
SATURATED FAT: 4G
CARBS: 51G
FIBER: 7G
SUGARS: 24G

SERVES

## Method

**↓ONE**
Ensure the motor base is fully charged. Install the blender cup on the base securely, then power on.

**↓TWO**
Add all the ingredients to the cup in **the order listed** (liquids followed by solids) ensuring the **max fill** line is not exceeded.

**↓THREE**
Secure the lid to the blender cup.

**↓FOUR**
Start the blending process. If necessary, repeat the blending process until completely smooth.

**↓FIVE**
Sip from the cup or pour into a glass and enjoy!

# COCONUT FLOUR SMOOTHIE

## Ingredients

→ **1 CUP UNSWEETENED COCONUT MILK**

→ **½ SMALL BANANA, CHOPPED**

→ **1 TBSP COCONUT FLOUR**

→ **1 TBSP CHIA SEEDS**

→ **½ TSP GROUND CINNAMON**

→ **1 SCOOP (30G) VANILLA PROTEIN POWDER**

→ **4-5 ICE CUBES**

### Nutrition

**CALORIES:** 400
**PROTEIN:** 28G
**TOTAL FAT:** 20G
**SATURATED FAT:** 15G
**CARBS:** 35G
**FIBER:** 12G
**SUGARS:** 15G

**SERVES**

## Method

**↓ONE**
Ensure the motor base is fully charged. Install the blender cup on the base securely, then power on.

**↓TWO**
Add all the ingredients to the cup in **the order listed** (liquids followed by solids) ensuring the **max fill** line is not exceeded.

**↓THREE**
Secure the lid to the blender cup.

**↓FOUR**
Start the blending process. If necessary, repeat the blending process until completely smooth.

**↓FIVE**
Sip from the cup or pour into a glass and enjoy!

# PEANUT BUTTER BANANA PROTEIN BLAST

## Ingredients

→ **1 CUP UNSWEETENED SOY MILK**

→ **½ SMALL BANANA, CHOPPED**

→ **¼ CUP ROLLED OATS**

→ **2 TBSP PEANUT BUTTER**

→ **1 TBSP CHIA SEEDS**

→ **4-5 ICE CUBES**

## Method

**↓ONE**
Ensure the motor base is fully charged. Install the blender cup on the base securely, then power on.

**↓TWO**
Add all the ingredients to the cup in **the order listed** (liquids followed by solids) ensuring the **max fill** line is not exceeded.

**↓THREE**
Secure the lid to the blender cup.

**↓FOUR**
Start the blending process. If necessary, repeat the blending process until completely smooth.

**↓FIVE**
Sip from the cup or pour into a glass and enjoy!

### Nutrition
CALORIES: 500
PROTEIN: 25G
TOTAL FAT: 24G
SATURATED FAT: 2.5G
CARBS: 52G
FIBER: 9G
SUGARS: 20G

SERVES

**1**

# BERRY GREEK YOGHURT SMOOTHIE

## Ingredients

→ **¾ CUP UNSWEETENED ALMOND MILK**

→ **½ CUP GREEK YOGURT**

→ **1 TBSP ALMOND BUTTER**

→ **1 TSP CHIA SEEDS**

→ **1 TBSP HONEY**

→ **⅓ CUP FROZEN RASPBERRIES**

→ **¼ CUP FROZEN BLACKBERRIES**

## Method

**↓ONE**
Ensure the motor base is fully charged. Install the blender cup on the base securely, then power on.

**↓TWO**
Add all the ingredients to the cup in **the order listed** (liquids followed by solids) ensuring the **max fill** line is not exceeded.

**↓THREE**
Secure the lid to the blender cup.

**↓FOUR**
Start the blending process. If necessary, repeat the blending process until completely smooth.

**↓FIVE**
Sip from the cup or pour into a glass and enjoy!

### Nutrition

CALORIES: 400
PROTEIN: 20G
TOTAL FAT: 22G
SATURATED FAT: 3G
CARBS: 38G
FIBER: 11G
SUGARS: 34G

SERVES

**1**

# CHOCOLATE PEANUT BUTTER PROTEIN SHAKE

## Ingredients

→ **1 CUP UNSWEETENED COCONUT MILK**

→ **½ SMALL BANANA, CHOPPED**

→ **2 TBSP PEANUT BUTTER**

→ **1 TBSP COCOA POWDER**

→ **1 SCOOP (30G) CHOCOLATE WHEY PROTEIN POWDER**

→ **4-5 ICE CUBES**

### Nutrition ~

CALORIES: 415
PROTEIN: 35G
TOTAL FAT: 24G
SATURATED FAT: 5G
CARBS: 27G
FIBER: 8G
SUGARS: 13G

**SERVES**

## Method

**↓ONE**
Ensure the motor base is fully charged. Install the blender cup on the base securely, then power on.

**↓TWO**
Add all the ingredients to the cup in **the order listed** (liquids followed by solids) ensuring the **max fill** line is not exceeded.

**↓THREE**
Secure the lid to the blender cup.

**↓FOUR**
Start the blending process. If necessary, repeat the blending process until completely smooth.

**↓FIVE**
Sip from the cup or pour into a glass and enjoy!

# GREEN PROTEIN MACHINE

## Ingredients

→ **1 CUP UNSWEETENED COCONUT MILK**

→ **½ AVOCADO, PITTED**

→ **HANDFUL KALE**

→ **1 TBSP CHIA SEEDS**

→ **1 SCOOP (30G) UNFLAVORED WHEY PROTEIN POWDER**

→ **½ CUP FROZEN MANGO CHUNKS**

### Nutrition

CALORIES: 380
PROTEIN: 28G
TOTAL FAT: 17G
SATURATED FAT: 4G
CARBS: 31G
FIBER: 13G
SUGARS: 18G

**SERVES**

1

## Method

**↓ONE**
Ensure the motor base is fully charged. Install the blender cup on the base securely, then power on.

**↓TWO**
Add all the ingredients to the cup in **the order listed** (liquids followed by solids) ensuring the **max fill** line is not exceeded.

**↓THREE**
Secure the lid to the blender cup.

**↓FOUR**
Start the blending process. If necessary, repeat the blending process until completely smooth.

**↓FIVE**
Sip from the cup or pour into a glass and enjoy!

# STRAWBERRY COTTAGE CHEESE SMOOTHIE

## Ingredients

→ **¾ CUP UNSWEETENED OAT MILK**

→ **½ TSP VANILLA EXTRACT**

→ **½ CUP COTTAGE CHEESE**

→ **1 TBSP HONEY**

→ **½ CUP FROZEN STRAWBERRIES**

## Method

**↓ONE**
Ensure the motor base is fully charged. Install the blender cup on the base securely, then power on.

**↓TWO**
Add all the ingredients to the cup in **the order listed** (liquids followed by solids) ensuring the **max fill** line is not exceeded.

**↓THREE**
Secure the lid to the blender cup.

**↓FOUR**
Start the blending process. If necessary, repeat the blending process until completely smooth.

**↓FIVE**
Sip from the cup or pour into a glass and enjoy!

### Nutrition ~
CALORIES: 310
PROTEIN: 24G
TOTAL FAT: 7G
SATURATED FAT: 2G
CARBS: 43G
FIBER: 2G
SUGARS: 37G

SERVES

1

# VANILLA ALMOND BUTTER PROTEIN SMOOTHIE

## Ingredients

→ **1 CUP UNSWEETENED ALMOND MILK**

→ **1 TSP VANILLA EXTRACT**

→ **½ SMALL BANANA, CHOPPED**

→ **2 TBSP ALMOND BUTTER**

→ **1 SCOOP (30G) VANILLA WHEY PROTEIN POWDER**

→ **4-5 ICE CUBES**

### Nutrition

**CALORIES: 420**
**PROTEIN: 34G**
**TOTAL FAT: 22G**
**SATURATED FAT: 1.5G**
**CARBS: 27G**
**FIBER: 6G**
**SUGARS: 16G**

**SERVES**

1

## Method

**↓ONE**
Ensure the motor base is fully charged. Install the blender cup on the base securely, then power on.

**↓TWO**
Add all the ingredients to the cup in **the order listed** (liquids followed by solids) ensuring the **max fill** line is not exceeded.

**↓THREE**
Secure the lid to the blender cup.

**↓FOUR**
Start the blending process. If necessary, repeat the blending process until completely smooth.

**↓FIVE**
Sip from the cup or pour into a glass and enjoy!

# TOFU BERRY PROTEIN SMOOTHIE

## Ingredients

→ **1 CUP UNSWEETENED SOY MILK**

→ **½ CUP SILKEN TOFU**

→ **1 TBSP HONEY**

→ **1 TBSP CHIA SEEDS**

→ **½ CUP MIXED BERRIES**

## Method

**↓ONE**
Ensure the motor base is fully charged. Install the blender cup on the base securely, then power on.

**↓TWO**
Add all the ingredients to the cup in **the order listed** (liquids followed by solids) ensuring the **max fill** line is not exceeded.

**↓THREE**
Secure the lid to the blender cup.

**↓FOUR**
Start the blending process. If necessary, repeat the blending process until completely smooth.

**↓FIVE**
Sip from the cup or pour into a glass and enjoy!

### Nutrition

CALORIES: 320
PROTEIN: 22G
TOTAL FAT: 12G
SATURATED FAT: 1.5G
CARBS: 35G
FIBER: 10G
SUGARS: 24G

SERVES

**1**

# COFFEE PROTEIN SHAKE

## Ingredients

→ **1 CUP UNSWEETENED OAT MILK**

→ **½ CUP COLD BREW COFFEE**

→ **1 TBSP ALMOND BUTTER**

→ **½ TSP CINNAMON**

→ **1 SCOOP (30G) VANILLA WHEY PROTEIN POWDER**

→ **4-5 ICE CUBES**

## Method

**↓ONE**
Ensure the motor base is fully charged. Install the blender cup on the base securely, then power on.

**↓TWO**
Add all the ingredients to the cup in **the order listed** (liquids followed by solids) ensuring the **max fill** line is not exceeded.

**↓THREE**
Secure the lid to the blender cup.

**↓FOUR**
Start the blending process. If necessary, repeat the blending process until completely smooth.

**↓FIVE**
Sip from the cup or pour into a glass and enjoy!

### Nutrition

CALORIES: 340
PROTEIN: 35G
TOTAL FAT: 16G
SATURATED FAT: 1.5G
CARBS: 17G
FIBER: 4G
SUGARS: 6G

SERVES

# MANGO HEMP PROTEIN SMOOTHIE

## Ingredients

→ **1 CUP UNSWEETENED COCONUT MILK**

→ **¼ CUP GREEK YOGURT**

→ **1 TBSP LIME JUICE**

→ **1 ORANGE, PEELED**

→ **1 TBSP HEMP SEEDS**

→ **½ CUP FROZEN MANGO CHUNKS**

### Nutrition ~

**CALORIES: 290**
**PROTEIN: 13G**
**TOTAL FAT: 9G**
**SATURATED FAT: 4G**
**CARBS: 45G**
**FIBER: 6G**
**SUGARS: 37G**

**SERVES**

## Method

**↓ONE**
Ensure the motor base is fully charged. Install the blender cup on the base securely, then power on.

**↓TWO**
Add all the ingredients to the cup in **the order listed** (liquids followed by solids) ensuring the **max fill** line is not exceeded.

**↓THREE**
Secure the lid to the blender cup.

**↓FOUR**
Start the blending process. If necessary, repeat the blending process until completely smooth.

**↓FIVE**
Sip from the cup or pour into a glass and enjoy!

# CHOCOLATE BANANA OATMEAL SMOOTHIE

## Ingredients

→ **1 CUP UNSWEETENED COCONUT MILK**

→ **½ SMALL BANANA, CHOPPED**

→ **¼ CUP ROLLED OATS**

→ **1 TBSP ALMOND BUTTER**

→ **1 TBSP COCOA POWDER**

→ **4-5 ICE CUBES**

### Nutrition

CALORIES: 415
PROTEIN: 12G
TOTAL FAT: 23G
SATURATED FAT: 10G
CARBS: 46G
FIBER: 10G
SUGARS: 18G

SERVES

## Method

**↓ONE**
Ensure the motor base is fully charged. Install the blender cup on the base securely, then power on.

**↓TWO**
Add all the ingredients to the cup in **the order listed** (liquids followed by solids) ensuring the **max fill** line is not exceeded.

**↓THREE**
Secure the lid to the blender cup.

**↓FOUR**
Start the blending process. If necessary, repeat the blending process until completely smooth.

**↓FIVE**
Sip from the cup or pour into a glass and enjoy!

## PROTEIN

# BLUEBERRY MACA PROTEIN SMOOTHIE

## Ingredients

→ **1 CUP UNSWEETENED ALMOND MILK**

→ **1 TBSP LEMON JUICE**

→ **1 TBSP CHIA SEEDS**

→ **1 TSP MACA POWDER**

→ **1 SCOOP (30G) VANILLA WHEY PROTEIN POWDER**

→ **½ CUP FROZEN BLUEBERRIES**

### Nutrition

CALORIES: 280
PROTEIN: 30G
TOTAL FAT: 9G
SATURATED FAT: 1G
CARBS: 27G
FIBER: 8G
SUGARS: 15G

SERVES

## Method

**↓ONE**
Ensure the motor base is fully charged. Install the blender cup on the base securely, then power on.

**↓TWO**
Add all the ingredients to the cup in **the order listed** (liquids followed by solids) ensuring the **max fill** line is not exceeded.

**↓THREE**
Secure the lid to the blender cup.

**↓FOUR**
Start the blending process. If necessary, repeat the blending process until completely smooth.

**↓FIVE**
Sip from the cup or pour into a glass and enjoy!

## PROTEIN

# PEACH GINGER PROTEIN SMOOTHIE

## Ingredients

→ **1 CUP UNSWEETENED OAT MILK**

→ **1 TSP FRESHLY GRATED GINGER**

→ **1 TBSP ALMOND BUTTER**

→ **1 SCOOP (30G) UNFLAVORED WHEY PROTEIN POWDER**

→ **½ CUP FROZEN PEACH SLICES**

### Nutrition

CALORIES: 340
PROTEIN: 31G
TOTAL FAT: 16G
SATURATED FAT: 1.5G
CARBS: 22G
FIBER: 5G
SUGARS: 13G

**SERVES**

## Method

**↓ONE**
Ensure the motor base is fully charged. Install the blender cup on the base securely, then power on.

**↓TWO**
Add all the ingredients to the cup in **the order listed** (liquids followed by solids) ensuring the **max fill** line is not exceeded.

**↓THREE**
Secure the lid to the blender cup.

**↓FOUR**
Start the blending process. If necessary, repeat the blending process until completely smooth.

**↓FIVE**
Sip from the cup or pour into a glass and enjoy!

# AVOCADO SPINACH PROTEIN SMOOTHIE

## Ingredients

→ **1 CUP UNSWEETENED COCONUT MILK**

→ **1 TBSP LIME JUICE**

→ **HANDFUL SPINACH**

→ **½ AVOCADO, PITTED**

→ **1 SCOOP (30G) UNFLAVORED WHEY PROTEIN POWDER**

→ **4-5 ICE CUBES**

### Nutrition ~

CALORIES: 290
PROTEIN: 26G
TOTAL FAT: 15G
SATURATED FAT: 3G
CARBS: 15G
FIBER: 8G
SUGARS: 5G

SERVES

**1**

## Method

**↓ONE**
Ensure the motor base is fully charged. Install the blender cup on the base securely, then power on.

**↓TWO**
Add all the ingredients to the cup in **the order listed** (liquids followed by solids) ensuring the **max fill** line is not exceeded.

**↓THREE**
Secure the lid to the blender cup.

**↓FOUR**
Start the blending process. If necessary, repeat the blending process until completely smooth.

**↓FIVE**
Sip from the cup or pour into a glass and enjoy!

## PROTEIN

# BANANA FLAXSEED PROTEIN SMOOTHIE

## Ingredients

→ **1 CUP UNSWEETENED SOY MILK**

→ **1 TSP HONEY**

→ **½ SMALL BANANA, CHOPPED**

→ **½ TSP CINNAMON**

→ **1 TBSP GROUND FLAXSEED**

→ **1 SCOOP (30G) VANILLA WHEY PROTEIN POWDER**

→ **4-5 ICE CUBES**

### Nutrition

CALORIES: 400
PROTEIN: 39G
TOTAL FAT: 13G
SATURATED FAT: 1.5G
CARBS: 34G
FIBER: 6G
SUGARS: 26G

**SERVES**

1

## Method

**↓ONE**
Ensure the motor base is fully charged. Install the blender cup on the base securely, then power on.

**↓TWO**
Add all the ingredients to the cup in **the order listed** (liquids followed by solids) ensuring the **max fill** line is not exceeded.

**↓THREE**
Secure the lid to the blender cup.

**↓FOUR**
Start the blending process. If necessary, repeat the blending process until completely smooth.

**↓FIVE**
Sip from the cup or pour into a glass and enjoy!

# PROTEIN

# CHOCOLATE CHERRY PROTEIN SMOOTHIE

## Ingredients

→ **1 CUP UNSWEETENED ALMOND MILK**

→ **1 TBSP CHIA SEEDS**

→ **1 TBSP COCOA POWDER**

→ **1 SCOOP (30G) CHOCOLATE WHEY PROTEIN POWDER**

→ **½ CUP FROZEN PITTED CHERRIES**

### Nutrition
**CALORIES:** 330
**PROTEIN:** 32G
**TOTAL FAT:** 13G
**SATURATED FAT:** 3G
**CARBS:** 31G
**FIBER:** 10G
**SUGARS:** 15G

**SERVES**

1

## Method

**↓ONE**
Ensure the motor base is fully charged. Install the blender cup on the base securely, then power on.

**↓TWO**
Add all the ingredients to the cup in **the order listed** (liquids followed by solids) ensuring the **max fill** line is not exceeded.

**↓THREE**
Secure the lid to the blender cup.

**↓FOUR**
Start the blending process. If necessary, repeat the blending process until completely smooth.

**↓FIVE**
Sip from the cup or pour into a glass and enjoy!

GREEN

# SPINACH MANGO SMOOTHIE

## Ingredients

→ **1 CUP UNSWEETENED ALMOND MILK**

→ **1 TBSP LIME JUICE**

→ **½ SMALL BANANA, CHOPPED**

→ **½ MANGO FLESH PEELED & CHOPPED**

→ **HANDFUL SPINACH**

→ **1 TSP HONEY**

### Nutrition

CALORIES: 210
PROTEIN: 5G
TOTAL FAT: 7G
SATURATED FAT: 1G
CARBS: 38G
FIBER: 5G
SUGARS: 28G

SERVES

## Method

**↓ONE**
Ensure the motor base is fully charged. Install the blender cup on the base securely, then power on.

**↓TWO**
Add all the ingredients to the cup in **the order listed** (liquids followed by solids) ensuring the **max fill** line is not exceeded.

**↓THREE**
Secure the lid to the blender cup.

**↓FOUR**
Start the blending process. If necessary, repeat the blending process until completely smooth.

**↓FIVE**
Sip from the cup or pour into a glass and enjoy!

## GREEN

# CUCUMBER AVOCADO SMOOTHIE

## Ingredients

→ **1 CUP UNSWEETENED OAT MILK**

→ **1 TBSP LIME JUICE**

→ **½ AVOCADO, PITTED**

→ **⅓ CUCUMBER, CHOPPED**

→ **HANDFUL KALE**

→ **1 TSP CHIA SEEDS**

## Method

**↓ONE**
Ensure the motor base is fully charged. Install the blender cup on the base securely, then power on.

**↓TWO**
Add all the ingredients to the cup in **the order listed** (liquids followed by solids) ensuring the **max fill** line is not exceeded.

**↓THREE**
Secure the lid to the blender cup.

**↓FOUR**
Start the blending process. If necessary, repeat the blending process until completely smooth.

**↓FIVE**
Sip from the cup or pour into a glass and enjoy!

### Nutrition ~

CALORIES: 220
PROTEIN: 6G
TOTAL FAT: 12G
SATURATED FAT: 1.5G
CARBS: 26G
FIBER: 9G
SUGARS: 6G

**SERVES**

1

GREEN

# MATCHA PINEAPPLE SMOOTHIE

## Ingredients

→ **1 CUP UNSWEETENED COCONUT MILK**

→ **1 TBSP LEMON JUICE**

→ **HANDFUL SPINACH**

→ **1 TSP MATCHA POWDER**

→ **½ CUP FROZEN PINEAPPLE CHUNKS**

## Method

↓**ONE**
Ensure the motor base is fully charged. Install the blender cup on the base securely, then power on.

↓**TWO**
Add all the ingredients to the cup in **the order listed** (liquids followed by solids) ensuring the **max fill** line is not exceeded.

↓**THREE**
Secure the lid to the blender cup.

↓**FOUR**
Start the blending process. If necessary, repeat the blending process until completely smooth.

↓**FIVE**
Sip from the cup or pour into a glass and enjoy!

### Nutrition
CALORIES: 195
PROTEIN: 4G
TOTAL FAT: 5G
SATURATED FAT: 4G
CARBS: 37G
FIBER: 4G
SUGARS: 27G

SERVES

1

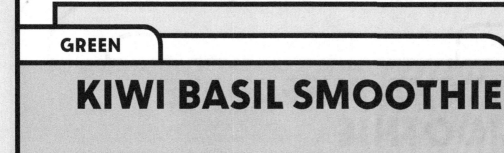

## GREEN

# KIWI BASIL SMOOTHIE

## Ingredients

→ **1 CUP UNSWEETENED SOY MILK**

→ **½ SMALL BANANA, CHOPPED**

→ **2 KIWIS, PEELED & CHOPPED**

→ **5 FRESH BASIL LEAVES**

→ **HANDFUL SPINACH**

→ **2-3 ICE CUBES**

## Method

**↓ONE**
Ensure the motor base is fully charged. Install the blender cup on the base securely, then power on.

**↓TWO**
Add all the ingredients to the cup in **the order listed** (liquids followed by solids) ensuring the **max fill** line is not exceeded.

**↓THREE**
Secure the lid to the blender cup.

**↓FOUR**
Start the blending process. If necessary, repeat the blending process until completely smooth.

**↓FIVE**
Sip from the cup or pour into a glass and enjoy!

### Nutrition

**CALORIES:** 250
**PROTEIN:** 13G
**TOTAL FAT:** 8G
**SATURATED FAT:** 1G
**CARBS:** 36G
**FIBER:** 6G
**SUGARS:** 27G

**SERVES**

1

## GREEN

# MINT KALE SMOOTHIE

## Ingredients

→ **1 CUP UNSWEETENED SOY MILK**

→ **1 TBSP LIME JUICE**

→ **⅓ CUCUMBER, CHOPPED**

→ **10 FRESH MINT LEAVES**

→ **HANDFUL KALE**

→ **2 TSP HONEY**

### Nutrition
CALORIES: 120
PROTEIN: 8G
TOTAL FAT: 3G
SATURATED FAT: 0G
CARBS: 18G
FIBER: 4G
SUGARS: 10G

SERVES

## Method

**↓ONE**
Ensure the motor base is fully charged. Install the blender cup on the base securely, then power on.

**↓TWO**
Add all the ingredients to the cup in **the order listed** (liquids followed by solids) ensuring the **max fill** line is not exceeded.

**↓THREE**
Secure the lid to the blender cup.

**↓FOUR**
Start the blending process. If necessary, repeat the blending process until completely smooth.

**↓FIVE**
Sip from the cup or pour into a glass and enjoy!

## GREEN

# AVOCADO CILANTRO SMOOTHIE

## Ingredients

→ **1 CUP UNSWEETENED ALMOND MILK**

→ **1 TBSP LIME JUICE**

→ **½ AVOCADO, PITTED**

→ **½ GREEN APPLE, CORED & CHOPPED**

→ **10 FRESH CILANTRO LEAVES**

→ **HANDFUL SPINACH**

→ **1 TSP HONEY**

### Nutrition

CALORIES: 290
PROTEIN: 4G
TOTAL FAT: 22G
SATURATED FAT: 3G
CARBS: 24G
FIBER: 10G
SUGARS: 13G

SERVES

## Method

**↓ONE**
Ensure the motor base is fully charged. Install the blender cup on the base securely, then power on.

**↓TWO**
Add all the ingredients to the cup in **the order listed** (liquids followed by solids) ensuring the **max fill** line is not exceeded.

**↓THREE**
Secure the lid to the blender cup.

**↓FOUR**
Start the blending process. If necessary, repeat the blending process until completely smooth.

**↓FIVE**
Sip from the cup or pour into a glass and enjoy!

# KIWI SPINACH SMOOTHIE

## Ingredients

→ **1 CUP UNSWEETENED OAT MILK**

→ **1 TBSP LEMON JUICE**

→ **½ SMALL BANANA, CHOPPED**

→ **2 KIWIS, PEELED & CHOPPED**

→ **HANDFUL SPINACH**

## Method

**↓ONE**
Ensure the motor base is fully charged. Install the blender cup on the base securely, then power on.

**↓TWO**
Add all the ingredients to the cup in **the order listed** (liquids followed by solids) ensuring the **max fill** line is not exceeded.

**↓THREE**
Secure the lid to the blender cup.

**↓FOUR**
Start the blending process. If necessary, repeat the blending process until completely smooth.

**↓FIVE**
Sip from the cup or pour into a glass and enjoy!

### Nutrition ～
CALORIES: 230
PROTEIN: 5G
TOTAL FAT: 4G
SATURATED FAT: 0.5G
CARBS: 43G
FIBER: 7G
SUGARS: 26G

SERVES

1

**GREEN**

# CUCUMBER PARSLEY SMOOTHIE

## Ingredients

→ **1 CUP UNSWEETENED COCONUT MILK**

→ **1 TBSP LEMON JUICE**

→ **⅓ CUCUMBER, CHOPPED**

→ **½ GREEN APPLE, CORED & CHOPPED**

→ **2 TSP FRESH PARSLEY LEAVES**

→ **HANDFUL KALE**

## Method

**↓ONE**
Ensure the motor base is fully charged. Install the blender cup on the base securely, then power on.

**↓TWO**
Add all the ingredients to the cup in **the order listed** (liquids followed by solids) ensuring the **max fill** line is not exceeded.

**↓THREE**
Secure the lid to the blender cup.

**↓FOUR**
Start the blending process. If necessary, repeat the blending process until completely smooth.

**↓FIVE**
Sip from the cup or pour into a glass and enjoy!

### Nutrition
**CALORIES:** 240
**PROTEIN:** 5G
**TOTAL FAT:** 5G
**SATURATED FAT:** 4G
**CARBS:** 46G
**FIBER:** 7G
**SUGARS:** 34G

**SERVES**

1

## GREEN

# MATCHA KIWI SMOOTHIE

## Ingredients

→ **1 CUP UNSWEETENED SOY MILK**

→ **1 TBSP LIME JUICE**

→ **½ SMALL BANANA, CHOPPED**

→ **1 KIWI, PEELED & CHOPPED**

→ **1 TSP MATCHA POWDER**

→ **HANDFUL SPINACH**

### Nutrition

CALORIES: 240
PROTEIN: 10G
TOTAL FAT: 8G
SATURATED FAT: 1G
CARBS: 37G
FIBER: 7G
SUGARS: 22G

**SERVES**

## Method

**↓ONE**
Ensure the motor base is fully charged. Install the blender cup on the base securely, then power on.

**↓TWO**
Add all the ingredients to the cup in **the order listed** (liquids followed by solids) ensuring the **max fill** line is not exceeded.

**↓THREE**
Secure the lid to the blender cup.

**↓FOUR**
Start the blending process. If necessary, repeat the blending process until completely smooth.

**↓FIVE**
Sip from the cup or pour into a glass and enjoy!

# GREEN

# AVOCADO KALE SMOOTHIE

## Ingredients

→ **1 CUP UNSWEETENED ALMOND MILK**

→ **¼ CUP GREEK YOGURT**

→ **½ AVOCADO, PITTED**

→ **HANDFUL KALE**

→ **1 TSP CHIA SEEDS**

→ **1 TSP HONEY**

### Nutrition

**CALORIES:** 380
**PROTEIN:** 14G
**TOTAL FAT:** 27G
**SATURATED FAT:** 3.5G
**CARBS:** 28G
**FIBER:** 13G
**SUGARS:** 11G

**SERVES**

## Method

**↓ONE**
Ensure the motor base is fully charged. Install the blender cup on the base securely, then power on.

**↓TWO**
Add all the ingredients to the cup in **the order listed** (liquids followed by solids) ensuring the **max fill** line is not exceeded.

**↓THREE**
Secure the lid to the blender cup.

**↓FOUR**
Start the blending process. If necessary, repeat the blending process until completely smooth.

**↓FIVE**
Sip from the cup or pour into a glass and enjoy!

# GREEN

# SPINACH DILL SMOOTHIE

## Ingredients

→ **1 CUP UNSWEETENED OAT MILK**

→ **1 TBSP LIME JUICE**

→ **½ GREEN APPLE, CORED & CHOPPED**

→ **5 FRESH DILL SPRIGS**

→ **HANDFUL SPINACH**

## Method

**↓ONE**
Ensure the motor base is fully charged. Install the blender cup on the base securely, then power on.

**↓TWO**
Add all the ingredients to the cup in **the order listed** (liquids followed by solids) ensuring the **max fill** line is not exceeded.

**↓THREE**
Secure the lid to the blender cup.

**↓FOUR**
Start the blending process. If necessary, repeat the blending process until completely smooth.

**↓FIVE**
Sip from the cup or pour into a glass and enjoy!

### Nutrition
CALORIES: 130
PROTEIN: 5G
TOTAL FAT: 3G
SATURATED FAT: 0G
CARBS: 24G
FIBER: 5G
SUGARS: 13G

SERVES

1

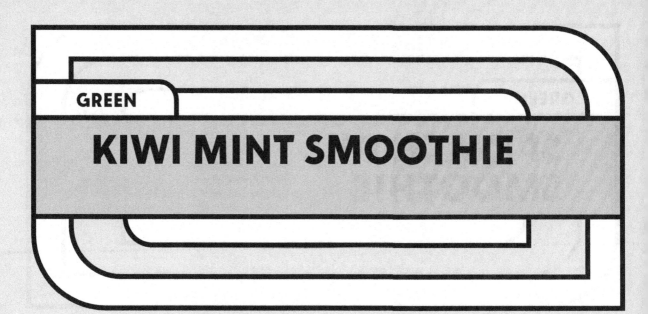

# GREEN

# KIWI MINT SMOOTHIE

## Ingredients

→ **1 CUP UNSWEETENED COCONUT MILK**

→ **1 TBSP LEMON JUICE**

→ **½ SMALL BANANA, CHOPPED**

→ **2 KIWIS, PEELED & CHOPPED**

→ **10 FRESH MINT LEAVES**

→ **HANDFUL SPINACH**

### Nutrition

CALORIES: 270
PROTEIN: 5G
TOTAL FAT: 5G
SATURATED FAT: 4G
CARBS: 58G
FIBER: 8G
SUGARS: 41G

**SERVES**

1

## Method

**↓ONE**
Ensure the motor base is fully charged. Install the blender cup on the base securely, then power on.

**↓TWO**
Add all the ingredients to the cup in **the order listed** (liquids followed by solids) ensuring the **max fill** line is not exceeded.

**↓THREE**
Secure the lid to the blender cup.

**↓FOUR**
Start the blending process. If necessary, repeat the blending process until completely smooth.

**↓FIVE**
Sip from the cup or pour into a glass and enjoy!

# GREEN

# CUCUMBER BASIL SMOOTHIE

## Ingredients

→ **1 CUP UNSWEETENED ALMOND MILK**

→ **1 TBSP LIME JUICE**

→ **⅓ CUCUMBER, CHOPPED**

→ **½ GREEN APPLE, CORED & CHOPPED**

→ **5 FRESH BASIL LEAVES**

→ **HANDFUL KALE**

## Method

**↓ONE**
Ensure the motor base is fully charged. Install the blender cup on the base securely, then power on.

**↓TWO**
Add all the ingredients to the cup in **the order listed** (liquids followed by solids) ensuring the **max fill** line is not exceeded.

**↓THREE**
Secure the lid to the blender cup.

**↓FOUR**
Start the blending process. If necessary, repeat the blending process until completely smooth.

**↓FIVE**
Sip from the cup or pour into a glass and enjoy!

### Nutrition
CALORIES: 190
PROTEIN: 5G
TOTAL FAT: 8G
SATURATED FAT: 1G
CARBS: 27G
FIBER: 6G
SUGARS: 16G

SERVES

1

**GREEN**

# AVOCADO PARSLEY SMOOTHIE

## Ingredients

→ **1 CUP UNSWEETENED SOY MILK**

→ **1 TBSP LEMON JUICE**

→ **½ AVOCADO, PITTED**

→ **½ SMALL BANANA, CHOPPED**

→ **2 TSP FRESH PARSLEY LEAVES**

→ **HANDFUL SPINACH**

### Nutrition ~
CALORIES: 290
PROTEIN: 12G
TOTAL FAT: 16G
SATURATED FAT: 2G
CARBS: 31G
FIBER: 11G
SUGARS: 13G

**SERVES**

**1**

## Method

**↓ONE**
Ensure the motor base is fully charged. Install the blender cup on the base securely, then power on.

**↓TWO**
Add all the ingredients to the cup in **the order listed** (liquids followed by solids) ensuring the **max fill** line is not exceeded.

**↓THREE**
Secure the lid to the blender cup.

**↓FOUR**
Start the blending process. If necessary, repeat the blending process until completely smooth.

**↓FIVE**
Sip from the cup or pour into a glass and enjoy!

## GREEN

# MATCHA SPINACH SMOOTHIE

## Ingredients

→ **1 CUP UNSWEETENED OAT MILK**

→ **1 TBSP LIME JUICE**

→ **½ SMALL BANANA, CHOPPED**

→ **HANDFUL SPINACH**

→ **1 TSP MATCHA POWDER**

→ **1 TSP HONEY**

## Method

**↓ONE**
Ensure the motor base is fully charged. Install the blender cup on the base securely, then power on.

**↓TWO**
Add all the ingredients to the cup in **the order listed** (liquids followed by solids) ensuring the **max fill** line is not exceeded.

**↓THREE**
Secure the lid to the blender cup.

**↓FOUR**
Start the blending process. If necessary, repeat the blending process until completely smooth.

**↓FIVE**
Sip from the cup or pour into a glass and enjoy!

### Nutrition

CALORIES: 210
PROTEIN: 5G
TOTAL FAT: 4G
SATURATED FAT: 0.5G
CARBS: 40G
FIBER: 5G
SUGARS: 26G

SERVES

# CINNAMON APPLE SMOOTHIE

## Ingredients

→ **1 CUP UNSWEETENED SOY MILK**

→ **1 GREEN APPLE, CORED & CHOPPED**

→ **1 TBSP ALMOND BUTTER**

→ **1 TSP GROUND CINNAMON**

→ **4-5 ICE CUBES**

## Method

### ↓ONE
Ensure the motor base is fully charged. Install the blender cup on the base securely, then power on.

### ↓TWO
Add all the ingredients to the cup in **the order listed** (liquids followed by solids) ensuring the **max fill** line is not exceeded.

### ↓THREE
Secure the lid to the blender cup.

### ↓FOUR
Start the blending process. If necessary, repeat the blending process until completely smooth.

### ↓FIVE
Sip from the cup or pour into a glass and enjoy!

## Nutrition ~
**CALORIES: 280**
**PROTEIN: 10G**
**TOTAL FAT: 12G**
**SATURATED FAT: 1.5G**
**CARBS: 36G**
**FIBER: 7G**
**SUGARS: 24G**

**SERVES**

**1**

# BLACKBERRY BASIL SMOOTHIE

## Ingredients

→ **1 CUP UNSWEETENED ALMOND MILK**

→ **1 TSP LIME JUICE**

→ **½ SMALL BANANA, CHOPPED**

→ **5-6 FRESH BASIL LEAVES**

→ **1 TBSP CHIA SEEDS**

→ **½ CUP FROZEN BLACKBERRIES**

## Method

**↓ONE**
Ensure the motor base is fully charged. Install the blender cup on the base securely, then power on.

**↓TWO**
Add all the ingredients to the cup in **the order listed** (liquids followed by solids) ensuring the **max fill** line is not exceeded.

**↓THREE**
Secure the lid to the blender cup.

**↓FOUR**
Start the blending process. If necessary, repeat the blending process until completely smooth.

**↓FIVE**
Sip from the cup or pour into a glass and enjoy!

### Nutrition
CALORIES: 220
PROTEIN: 6G
TOTAL FAT: 7G
SATURATED FAT: 0G
CARBS: 38G
FIBER: 11G
SUGARS: 18G

**SERVES**

1

# TROPICAL PAPAYA SMOOTHIE

## Ingredients

→ **1 CUP UNSWEETENED COCONUT MILK**

→ **1 TBSP LIME JUICE**

→ **⅔ CUP PAPAYA FLESH CUBED, SEEDS DISCARDED**

→ **½ MANGO FLESH PEELED AND CHOPPED**

→ **1 TBSP HEMP SEEDS**

→ **4-5 ICE CUBES**

### Nutrition

CALORIES: 210
PROTEIN: 4G
TOTAL FAT: 5G
SATURATED FAT: 1G
CARBS: 45G
FIBER: 5G
SUGARS: 36G

**SERVES**

## Method

**↓ONE**
Ensure the motor base is fully charged. Install the blender cup on the base securely, then power on.

**↓TWO**
Add all the ingredients to the cup in **the order listed** (liquids followed by solids) ensuring the **max fill** line is not exceeded.

**↓THREE**
Secure the lid to the blender cup.

**↓FOUR**
Start the blending process. If necessary, repeat the blending process until completely smooth.

**↓FIVE**
Sip from the cup or pour into a glass and enjoy!

# CHOCOLATE MINT SMOOTHIE

## Ingredients

→ **1 CUP UNSWEETENED SOY MILK**

→ **1 TSP VANILLA EXTRACT**

→ **½ SMALL BANANA, CHOPPED**

→ **2 TBSP COCOA POWDER**

→ **1 TBSP ALMOND BUTTER**

→ **5-6 FRESH MINT LEAVES**

→ **4-5 ICE CUBES**

### Nutrition

CALORIES: 340
PROTEIN: 13G
TOTAL FAT: 18G
SATURATED FAT: 2.5G
CARBS: 37G
FIBER: 8G
SUGARS: 19G

SERVES

1

## Method

**↓ONE**
Ensure the motor base is fully charged. Install the blender cup on the base securely, then power on.

**↓TWO**
Add all the ingredients to the cup in **the order listed** (liquids followed by solids) ensuring the **max fill** line is not exceeded.

**↓THREE**
Secure the lid to the blender cup.

**↓FOUR**
Start the blending process. If necessary, repeat the blending process until completely smooth.

**↓FIVE**
Sip from the cup or pour into a glass and enjoy!

# GINGER PEACH SMOOTHIE

## Ingredients

→ **1 CUP UNSWEETENED COCONUT MILK**

→ **1 TSP FRESH GINGER, GRATED**

→ **1 TBSP GROUND FLAXSEED**

→ **1 TSP MAPLE SYRUP**

→ **⅔ CUP FROZEN PEACH SLICES**

## Method

**↓ONE**
Ensure the motor base is fully charged. Install the blender cup on the base securely, then power on.

**↓TWO**
Add all the ingredients to the cup in **the order listed** (liquids followed by solids) ensuring the **max fill** line is not exceeded.

**↓THREE**
Secure the lid to the blender cup.

**↓FOUR**
Start the blending process. If necessary, repeat the blending process until completely smooth.

**↓FIVE**
Sip from the cup or pour into a glass and enjoy!

### Nutrition ~

CALORIES: 280
PROTEIN: 3G
TOTAL FAT: 5G
SATURATED FAT: 4G
CARBS: 59G
FIBER: 6G
SUGARS: 50G

**SERVES**

**1**

# SPINACH PINEAPPLE SMOOTHIE

## Ingredients

→ **1 CUP UNSWEETENED OAT MILK**

→ **1 TBSP LIME JUICE**

→ **1 CUP PINEAPPLE, CUBED**

→ **HANDFUL SPINACH**

→ **1 TBSP CHIA SEEDS**

→ **4-5 ICE CUBES**

## Method

**↓ONE**
Ensure the motor base is fully charged. Install the blender cup on the base securely, then power on.

**↓TWO**
Add all the ingredients to the cup in **the order listed** (liquids followed by solids) ensuring the **max fill** line is not exceeded.

**↓THREE**
Secure the lid to the blender cup.

**↓FOUR**
Start the blending process. If necessary, repeat the blending process until completely smooth.

**↓FIVE**
Sip from the cup or pour into a glass and enjoy!

### Nutrition ～
**CALORIES:** 200
**PROTEIN:** 6G
**TOTAL FAT:** 5G
**SATURATED FAT:** 0.5G
**CARBS:** 35G
**FIBER:** 8G
**SUGARS:** 19G

**SERVES**

1

**VEGAN & DAIRY FREE**

# BANANA WALNUT SMOOTHIE

## Ingredients

→ **1 CUP UNSWEETENED SOY MILK**

→ **1 SMALL BANANA, CHOPPED**

→ **2 TBSP ALMOND BUTTER**

→ **1 TBSP WALNUTS**

→ **1 TBSP COCOA POWDER**

→ **1 TSP CINNAMON**

→ **4-5 ICE CUBES**

### Nutrition ~
CALORIES: 410
PROTEIN: 13G
TOTAL FAT: 30G
SATURATED FAT: 2.5G
CARBS: 29G
FIBER: 7G
SUGARS: 16G

SERVES

## Method

**↓ONE**
Ensure the motor base is fully charged. Install the blender cup on the base securely, then power on.

**↓TWO**
Add all the ingredients to the cup in **the order listed** (liquids followed by solids) ensuring the **max fill** line is not exceeded.

**↓THREE**
Secure the lid to the blender cup.

**↓FOUR**
Start the blending process. If necessary, repeat the blending process until completely smooth.

**↓FIVE**
Sip from the cup or pour into a glass and enjoy!

# RASPBERRY BEET SMOOTHIE

## Ingredients

→ **1 CUP UNSWEETENED SOY MILK**

→ **1 TSP VANILLA EXTRACT**

→ **1 SMALL BEET, PEELED AND CHOPPED**

→ **1 TBSP ALMOND BUTTER**

→ **½ CUP FROZEN RASPBERRIES**

### Nutrition ~
CALORIES: 290
PROTEIN: 12G
TOTAL FAT: 14G
SATURATED FAT: 1.5G
CARBS: 32G
FIBER: 10G
SUGARS: 17G

SERVES

## Method

**↓ONE**
Ensure the motor base is fully charged. Install the blender cup on the base securely, then power on.

**↓TWO**
Add all the ingredients to the cup in **the order listed** (liquids followed by solids) ensuring the **max fill** line is not exceeded.

**↓THREE**
Secure the lid to the blender cup.

**↓FOUR**
Start the blending process. If necessary, repeat the blending process until completely smooth.

**↓FIVE**
Sip from the cup or pour into a glass and enjoy!

# PEAR GINGER SMOOTHIE

## Ingredients

→ **1 CUP UNSWEETENED ALMOND MILK**

→ **1 PEAR, CORED & CHOPPED**

→ **1 TSP FRESH GINGER, GRATED**

→ **1 TBSP HEMP SEEDS**

→ **1 TSP MAPLE SYRUP**

→ **4-5 ICE CUBES**

### Nutrition

CALORIES: 240
PROTEIN: 6G
TOTAL FAT: 10G
SATURATED FAT: 1G
CARBS: 35G
FIBER: 8G
SUGARS: 25G

**SERVES**

## Method

**↓ONE**
Ensure the motor base is fully charged. Install the blender cup on the base securely, then power on.

**↓TWO**
Add all the ingredients to the cup in **the order listed** (liquids followed by solids) ensuring the **max fill** line is not exceeded.

**↓THREE**
Secure the lid to the blender cup.

**↓FOUR**
Start the blending process. If necessary, repeat the blending process until completely smooth.

**↓FIVE**
Sip from the cup or pour into a glass and enjoy!

# BLUEBERRY KALE SMOOTHIE

## Ingredients

→ **1 CUP UNSWEETENED COCONUT MILK**

→ **1 TSP LEMON JUICE**

→ **HANDFUL KALE**

→ **1 TBSP CHIA SEEDS**

→ **½ CUP FROZEN BLUEBERRIES**

### Nutrition

CALORIES: 250
PROTEIN: 5G
TOTAL FAT: 6G
SATURATED FAT: 4G
CARBS: 49G
FIBER: 10G
SUGARS: 32G

SERVES

## Method

**↓ONE**
Ensure the motor base is fully charged. Install the blender cup on the base securely, then power on.

**↓TWO**
Add all the ingredients to the cup in **the order listed** (liquids followed by solids) ensuring the **max fill** line is not exceeded.

**↓THREE**
Secure the lid to the blender cup.

**↓FOUR**
Start the blending process. If necessary, repeat the blending process until completely smooth.

**↓FIVE**
Sip from the cup or pour into a glass and enjoy!

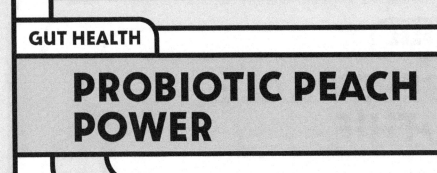

GUT HEALTH

# PROBIOTIC PEACH POWER

## Ingredients

→ **1 CUP PLAIN KEFIR**

→ **1 TBSP GROUND FLAXSEED**

→ **1 TBSP HONEY**

→ **½ TSP CINNAMON**

→ **⅔ CUP FROZEN PEACH SLICES**

## Method

**↓ONE**
Ensure the motor base is fully charged. Install the blender cup on the base securely, then power on.

**↓TWO**
Add all the ingredients to the cup in **the order listed** (liquids followed by solids) ensuring the **max fill** line is not exceeded.

**↓THREE**
Secure the lid to the blender cup.

**↓FOUR**
Start the blending process. If necessary, repeat the blending process until completely smooth.

**↓FIVE**
Sip from the cup or pour into a glass and enjoy!

### Nutrition

CALORIES: 330
PROTEIN: 12G
TOTAL FAT: 9G
SATURATED FAT: 2G
CARBS: 50G
FIBER: 4G
SUGARS: 41G

SERVES

# PREBIOTIC PINEAPPLE HEMP

## Ingredients

→ ¾ CUP GREEK YOGURT

→ ½ SMALL BANANA, CHOPPED

→ 2 TBSP ROLLED OATS

→ 1 TBSP HEMP SEEDS

→ ¾ CUP FROZEN PINEAPPLE CHUNKS

## Method

**↓ONE**
Ensure the motor base is fully charged. Install the blender cup on the base securely, then power on.

**↓TWO**
Add all the ingredients to the cup in **the order listed** (liquids followed by solids) ensuring the **max fill** line is not exceeded.

**↓THREE**
Secure the lid to the blender cup.

**↓FOUR**
Start the blending process. If necessary, repeat the blending process until completely smooth.

**↓FIVE**
Sip from the cup or pour into a glass and enjoy!

### Nutrition ～

CALORIES: 370
PROTEIN: 16G
TOTAL FAT: 11G
SATURATED FAT: 2G
CARBS: 57G
FIBER: 7G
SUGARS: 34G

SERVES

# CHERRY CHOCOLATE PROBIOTIC

## Ingredients

→ **1 CUP PLAIN KEFIR**

→ **2 TBSP DARK CHOCOLATE CHIPS**

→ **1 TBSP MAPLE SYRUP**

→ **¾ CUP FROZEN PITTED CHERRIES**

## Method

**↓ONE**
Ensure the motor base is fully charged. Install the blender cup on the base securely, then power on.

**↓TWO**
Add all the ingredients to the cup in **the order listed** (liquids followed by solids) ensuring the **max fill** line is not exceeded.

**↓THREE**
Secure the lid to the blender cup.

**↓FOUR**
Start the blending process. If necessary, repeat the blending process until completely smooth.

**↓FIVE**
Sip from the cup or pour into a glass and enjoy!

### Nutrition ~
**CALORIES:** 410
**PROTEIN:** 14G
**TOTAL FAT:** 15G
**SATURATED FAT:** 8G
**CARBS:** 56G
**FIBER:** 5G
**SUGARS:** 41G

SERVES

1

# GUT HEALTH

# PREBIOTIC GREEN DREAM

## Ingredients

→ **1 CUP NATURAL YOGURT**

→ **1 GREEN APPLE, CORED & CHOPPED**

→ **HANDFUL SPINACH**

→ **2 TBSP CHIA SEEDS**

→ **1 TBSP HONEY**

## Method

**↓ONE**
Ensure the motor base is fully charged. Install the blender cup on the base securely, then power on.

**↓TWO**
Add all the ingredients to the cup in **the order listed** (liquids followed by solids) ensuring the **max fill** line is not exceeded.

**↓THREE**
Secure the lid to the blender cup.

**↓FOUR**
Start the blending process. If necessary, repeat the blending process until completely smooth.

**↓FIVE**
Sip from the cup or pour into a glass and enjoy!

### Nutrition

CALORIES: 400
PROTEIN: 16G
TOTAL FAT: 12G
SATURATED FAT: 4G
CARBS: 59G
FIBER: 14G
SUGARS: 37G

SERVES

1

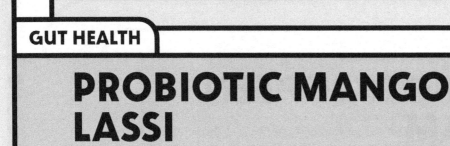

# PROBIOTIC MANGO LASSI

## Ingredients

→ **½ CUP UNSWEETENED ALMOND MILK**

→ **½ CUP GREEK YOGURT**

→ **1 TBSP LEMON JUICE**

→ **¼ TSP GROUND CARDAMOM**

→ **2 TBSP ROLLED OATS**

→ **½ CUP FROZEN MANGO CHUNKS**

### Nutrition ~

CALORIES: 290
PROTEIN: 10G
TOTAL FAT: 7G
SATURATED FAT: 1G
CARBS: 44G
FIBER: 5G
SUGARS: 29G

**SERVES**

## Method

**↓ONE**
Ensure the motor base is fully charged. Install the blender cup on the base securely, then power on.

**↓TWO**
Add all the ingredients to the cup in **the order listed** (liquids followed by solids) ensuring the **max fill** line is not exceeded.

**↓THREE**
Secure the lid to the blender cup.

**↓FOUR**
Start the blending process. If necessary, repeat the blending process until completely smooth.

**↓FIVE**
Sip from the cup or pour into a glass and enjoy!

# TROPICAL SUNSET SLUSHIE

## Ingredients

→ ¾ CUP PINEAPPLE JUICE

→ ½ CUP UNSWEETENED COCONUT MILK

→ ½ SMALL BANANA, CHOPPED

→ ½ CUP FROZEN MANGO CHUNKS

## Method

**↓ONE**
Ensure the motor base is fully charged. Install the blender cup on the base securely, then power on.

**↓TWO**
Add all the ingredients to the cup in **the order listed** (liquids followed by solids) ensuring the **max fill** line is not exceeded.

**↓THREE**
Secure the lid to the blender cup.

**↓FOUR**
Start the blending process. If necessary, repeat the blending process until completely smooth.

**↓FIVE**
Sip from the cup or pour into a glass and enjoy!

### Nutrition ~
CALORIES: 160
PROTEIN: 2G
TOTAL FAT: 1G
SATURATED FAT: OG
CARBS: 39G
FIBER: 3G
SUGARS: 32G

SERVES

1

# WATERMELON CUCUMBER COOLER

## Ingredients

→ **1 CUP UNSWEETENED COCONUT MILK**

→ **¾ CUP FRESH WATERMELON, CUBED**

→ **⅓ CUCUMBER, CHOPPED**

→ **4-5 FRESH MINT LEAVES**

→ **1 TBSP LIME JUICE**

→ **1 TSP FRESH GINGER, PEELED & GRATED**

→ **1 TSP HONEY**

→ **2-3 ICE CUBES**

### Nutrition

CALORIES: 80
PROTEIN: 1G
TOTAL FAT: 0G
SATURATED FAT: 0G
CARBS: 20G
FIBER: 1G
SUGARS: 17G

SERVES

## Method

**↓ONE**
Ensure the motor base is fully charged. Install the blender cup on the base securely, then power on.

**↓TWO**
Add all the ingredients to the cup in **the order listed** (liquids followed by solids) ensuring the **max fill** line is not exceeded.

**↓THREE**
Secure the lid to the blender cup.

**↓FOUR**
Start the blending process. If necessary, repeat the blending process until completely smooth.

**↓FIVE**
Sip from the cup or pour into a glass and enjoy!

# PINEAPPLE BASIL SLUSHIE

## Ingredients

→ **½ CUP PINEAPPLE JUICE**

→ **½ CUP UNSWEETENED COCONUT MILK**

→ **1 TBSP LIME JUICE**

→ **5-6 FRESH BASIL LEAVES**

→ **½ CUP FROZEN PINEAPPLE CHUNKS**

→ **2-3 ICE CUBES**

## Method

**↓ONE**
Ensure the motor base is fully charged. Install the blender cup on the base securely, then power on.

**↓TWO**
Add all the ingredients to the cup in **the order listed** (liquids followed by solids) ensuring the **max fill** line is not exceeded.

**↓THREE**
Secure the lid to the blender cup.

**↓FOUR**
Start the blending process. If necessary, repeat the blending process until completely smooth.

**↓FIVE**
Sip from the cup or pour into a glass and enjoy!

### Nutrition

CALORIES: 200
PROTEIN: 2G
TOTAL FAT: 7G
SATURATED FAT: 6G
CARBS: 38G
FIBER: 4G
SUGARS: 30G

**SERVES**

1

99

# PEACH MANGO TANGO SLUSHIE

## Ingredients

→ **½ CUP PEACH JUICE**

→ **½ CUP MANGO JUICE**

→ **¼ CUP FROZEN PEACH SLICES?**

→ **¼ CUP FROZEN MANGO CHUNKS?**

→ **2-3 ICE CUBES**

### Nutrition
**Calories:** 120
**Protein:** 1g
**Total Fat:** 0g
**Saturated Fat:** 0g
**Carbs:** 30g
**Fiber:** 2g
**Sugars:** 27g

**SERVES**

1

## Method

**↓ONE**
Ensure the motor base is fully charged. Install the blender cup on the base securely, then power on.

**↓TWO**
Add all the ingredients to the cup in **the order listed** (liquids followed by solids) ensuring the **max fill** line is not exceeded.

**↓THREE**
Secure the lid to the blender cup.

**↓FOUR**
Start the blending process. If necessary, repeat the blending process until completely smooth.

**↓FIVE**
Sip from the cup or pour into a glass and enjoy!

# STRAWBERRY GREEN TEA COOLER

## Ingredients

→ **1 CUP GREEN TEA, CHILLED**

→ **1 TBSP LEMON JUICE**

→ **1 TSP HONEY**

→ **½ CUP FROZEN STRAWBERRIES**

→ **2-3 ICE CUBES**

## Method

**↓ONE**
Ensure the motor base is fully charged. Install the blender cup on the base securely, then power on.

**↓TWO**
Add all the ingredients to the cup in **the order listed** (liquids followed by solids) ensuring the **max fill** line is not exceeded.

**↓THREE**
Secure the lid to the blender cup.

**↓FOUR**
Start the blending process. If necessary, repeat the blending process until completely smooth.

**↓FIVE**
Sip from the cup or pour into a glass and enjoy!

### Nutrition
CALORIES: 54
PROTEIN: 0G
TOTAL FAT: 0G
SATURATED FAT: 0G
CARBS: 14G
FIBER: 1G
SUGARS: 12G

SERVES

1

# Index

Made in the USA
Coppell, TX
28 March 2025

47638084R10057